Job
Burnout

Microcultures That Lead to a Low-stress Workplace

(How to Prevent Job Burnout and Get Your Enthusiasm for Work Back)

Fred Martin

Published By **Bella Frost**

Fred Martin

Job Burnout: Microcultures That Lead to a Low-stress Workplace (How to Prevent Job Burnout and Get Your Enthusiasm for Work Back)

ISBN   978-1-7775324-2-0

No part of this guidebook shall be reproduced in any form without permission in writing from the publisher except in the case of brief quotations embodied in critical articles or reviews.

Legal & Disclaimer

The information contained in this book is not designed to replace or take the place of any form of medicine or professional medical advice. The information in this book has been provided for educational & entertainment purposes only.

The information contained in this book has been compiled from sources deemed reliable, and it is accurate to the best of the Author's knowledge; however, the Author cannot guarantee its accuracy and validity and cannot be held liable for any errors or omissions. Changes are periodically made to this book. You must consult your doctor or get professional medical advice before using any of the suggested remedies, techniques, or information in this book.

Table Of Contents

Chapter 1: Understanding the 80 Hour Work Week 1

Chapter 2: Managing Your Time............. 11

Chapter 3: Managing Your Energy.......... 24

Chapter 4: Maintaining Your Health And Well-Being 32

Chapter 5: Managing Stress and Burnout50

Chapter 6: Achieving Success during the 80 Hour Work Week 60

Chapter 7: Understanding the Effects of Burnout... 81

Chapter 8: Signs and Symptoms of Burnout 88

Chapter 9: The Consequences of Ignoring Burnout... 96

Chapter 10: Strategies for Preventing Burnout... 101

Chapter 11: Strategies To Recover 116

Chapter 12: Creating a Sustainable Work-Life Balance.. 131

Chapter 13: Cultivating Resilience........ 139

Chapter 14: Finding Joy and Purpose ... 151

Chapter 15: Get Clarity Success, Different 163

Chapter 16: Who Are Curious Are Fascinating? 174

Chapter 1: Understanding the 80 Hour Work Week

In today's hectic work environment In today's fast-paced work environment, many professionals are in a long-term work schedule, depriving their time for personal enjoyment, and battling to achieve the balance of work and family. This is often referred to as the"80-hour" Work Week, and it could take a major physical and psychological burden on those who suffer from it.

What's the 80-hour Work Week?

There isn't a single definition for the term "80-hour" Work Week; it typically is a reference to schedules of work that demand employees to be working longer than 40 hours per week for a period of time. It could be in shape in the form of working longer hours in an office environment or having to be able to work from home or often travel in order to satisfy work requirements.

The typical 80-hour Work Week can vary in length and frequency, based on the company, industry as well as the individual requirements of each job sometimes, it might require employees to work longer hours over a brief period duration, like when the season is busy or when you need to meet a certain date. Sometimes it could be an everyday aspect of work, where employees are expected to endure for long hours on a regular or every week.

Why Do Some Jobs Require This Schedule?

There are a variety of reasons certain jobs demand employees to be on the job for long periods of time. In certain instances this could be due because of the nature work like the field of emergency or healthcare, which requires 24-hour care. Sometimes this could be because of a corporate one's culture which values working longer hours and regards these as an indication of commitment and dedication. No matter the reason that it is the case, an 80-hour Work Week can be challenging for people who have to endure it. It is essential to know the physical and mental strains that come with such a work routine.

Certain types of jobs that may require an 80-hour Week of Work Week

Extended hours at work are an everyday reality for many people working in today's busy and globalized world. Some jobs permit the typical nine-to-5 work timetable, some require an eight-hour workweek that includes fifty, sixty, or even a total of 80 hours every week. The following industries most of these positions need an hour-long working week.

Medical Professionals

Doctors, medical professionals as well as nurses and healthcare professionals are frequently called upon to work for long periods of time especially in emergency rooms and hospitals. Based on a research conducted from the National Institute for Occupational Safety and Health Medical professionals are employed on average between 50 and 60 hours a week. There are some specialty areas like surgery which require even more durations. A lot of people working in this field have a strong commitment to their jobs and are required to work for long hours to help their patients, and to satisfy the changing needs for their work.

Lawyers

Lawyers also are well-known for their lengthy hours, especially in big law firms. Based on a study conducted from the American Bar Association, lawyers who practice in private practice can expect to typically work 50 hours a week and some even work up to 80 hours a week during the peak times.

Investment Bankers

The investment bankers have a reputation for their long working hours, particularly in mergers and acquisitions as well as other deals that are high-stress. Based on a study conducted of Wall Street Oasis, investment bankers are employed for an average of 70 to

100 hours a week. Some of them work as much as 120 hours per week during peak hours.

Consultants

Consultants, especially those who specialize involved in management consulting are known to travel often and working long durations. According to research conducted from Consulting Magazine, consultants work on average 60 to 70 hours each week and some even work up to 80 hours per week in the peak times.

Entrepreneurs

Entrepreneurs, especially those who work operating in startups, usually have long working hours in order to create their business from the bottom starting from scratch. According to a research conducted of Startup Genome, startup founders typically work 60-80 hours per week. Some of them work more than 100 hours a week at the start of their business.

Why Do These Jobs Require an 80 Hour Work Week?

There are many reasons the jobs that require these types of positions need an hours of work per week. The reasons are diverse:

"High Demand Jobs such as medical specialists attorneys, investment bankers as well as consultants are highly sought-after, which is why they usually require a great deal of work to perform.

Deadlines: Jobs such as consultancy and investment banking often are characterized by deadlines that are tight, and requires employees to work lengthy days to make sure they meet the deadlines.

Needs of the client: The majority of these positions require working with clients who might require urgent assistance or have unexpected requirements that need to be addressed quickly.

The culture of startups Entrepreneurs typically work for long hours in order to start their business up and running and to build momentum. The long hours are now normal in the business culture.

Although an eight-hour working week might not suit everyone however, it is a common occurrence for some professionals working in certain fields. jobs like medical professionals, attorneys, investment bankers entrepreneurs and consultants typically have long working hours required to satisfy the demands of clients, deadlines as well as the high demands. If you're contemplating a career in any of these fields you must be ready of working long hours, and come up with strategies to reduce the stress of working, balancing work and life and reaching successful. If you have the proper equipment and tools will allow you to excel within these challenging professions and reach your goals in the workplace.

The Physical and Mental Toll of Long Work Weeks

Being in a long-term work environment regularly could have an effect on your physical and mental well-being. Research has shown that prolonged days at work are associated with an increased risk of developing chronic illnesses, such as diabetes, heart disease as well as obesity. Furthermore, working long week can result in increased stress depression, anxiety, and stress along with a decline in levels of satisfaction at work and the overall level of living.

The physical effects of an hours of the Work Week are well-documented. Working long hours may cause muscles strain and fatigue or even injuries. Being in a seated position for long times can raise the chance of developing muscle-skeletal issues, including carpal tunnel syndrome, or back discomfort. The psychological effects of the eight-hour Work Week can be just as important. Working long hours may result in increased anxiety and stress, which may affect your eating habits, sleep quality as well as overall health. Stress is connected to various ailments, like heart disease, depression, as well as stroke.

With the numerous well-documented issues with health that come from working an intense workweek and the stress of it, it is imperative for you to discover strategies to improve your working week, especially if you have a situation in which you are living a typical life the person you are.

How to manage the 80-hour Work Week

Due to the potential physical and mental strains that can be incurred by the 80-hour Work Week, it is essential to plan to control this working schedule efficiently. In the next chapters, we'll look at ways to use practical techniques and strategies to manage your time, remaining efficient and enthusiastic, keeping an appropriate balance between work and life and establishing strong bonds with colleagues and other employees, and so on.

Understanding the 80-hour Work Week and its potential effects, you'll be able to be in control of your working time and enjoy greater enjoyment and satisfaction both in your professional and the personal. If you're a professional who is busy or an entrepreneur, or any other person that works for in a long-term, sedentary schedule, this guide will provide all the information and tools you'll need to succeed in today's hectic working environment.

Chapter 2: Managing Your Time

One of the major problems of an 80-hour Work Week is managing your time efficiently. With so many obligations to meet it's difficult to organize your activities and focus on what's the most crucial. In this section we'll discuss some effective methods for managing time to ensure you are in control of your work as well as achieve more effectiveness and efficiency.

A well-planned and efficient time management system is essential in an 80-hour week. It will provide many benefits such as:

Improved productivity controlling your time efficiently You can prioritize your work and concentrate on the important tasks. This will allow you to perform more effectively and boost the overall efficiency, which allows you to complete more tasks within a shorter amount of time.

Reduced stress there's a lot of work of work to complete it's not difficult to get overloaded and stressed. A good time management system will help you remain organized and decrease stress levels because you'll have a clearly defined strategy for what has to be accomplished and at what time.

Improved balance between work and life: Long hours of work could make it challenging to achieve a balanced life-work equilibrium. A well-planned time management strategy helps you have additional time for leisure, which allows you to pursue activities, enjoy time with your loved ones as well as prioritize your mental and physical well-being.

Improved decision-making you're working long hours it's not uncommon to rush or make uninformed choices. Time management is a good tool to assist you in taking a look back and make better decisions because you'll be able to take into consideration all pertinent aspects.

A higher level of satisfaction with your job In the event that you are competent in managing your time well it's likely that you'll be feeling a sense of achievement and fulfillment as you check things off your list of to-dos. This will make to feel happier in your job and improve the overall satisfaction of your job.

Time Management Techniques

Time management that is effective is about identifying the strategies and tools that are most effective for your needs. Some common time management techniques include:

Making a list of things to do writing down the daily tasks can aid in staying focus and organized on the tasks that must be accomplished. If you're working for long hours you can easily forget crucial tasks, or get lost of what must be completed following. When you make a checklist of things to do it will help you stay in control of your work and be sure that you're working on the most crucial tasks.

Prioritizing your work: When you've compiled your to-do lists it is essential to set priorities for your work. This means determining the most critical tasks, and then tackling them first prior to moving onto lesser-important jobs. Prioritizing your projects ensures you're paying attention to the aspects which matter the most, and you're moving towards your goal.

Utilizing a timer: An efficient method to manage your time is by using the timer. Create a timer that is set for an amount of time like 25 minutes. You then perform a task until the timer is set. This method, also known as The Pomodoro Technique, can help keep you focused and eliminate distractions. When the timer is set and you're not in a hurry, stop for a moment before repeating the sequence.

The idea of breaking tasks down into smaller pieces When a project feels daunting, think about break it into manageable, smaller chunks. It can help keep you in the right mindset and stay focused to the work at hand. If, for instance, you're engaged in a large task, consider splitting it into a smaller task like researching, outlining and writing.

Planning out your time for certain activities: Create certain blocks of time to complete activities that demand your complete focus, like replying to emails or completing a task. If you block out time for those tasks, you'll be able to be sure you're focusing all your attention while working towards achieving your goals.

Prioritizing Your Tasks

One of the most important aspects for efficient time management is focusing on the tasks you have to complete. If you're faced with a lengthy to-do list, it could become easy to be overwhelmed and confused about the best place to begin. When you identify the most critical jobs and working on them prior to the others, you'll be able to be sure you're progressing in the areas which matter the most.

For effective prioritization of your work Try these actions:

Write down all your tasks that you must accomplish. This could be the tasks related to work and personal duties.

Determine the jobs which are the most crucial or that have the shortest date. These could be tasks which are crucial for your work or with a deadline.

Sort your work in the order they are important. It is important to determine which projects require the most attention or are crucial or urgent, and could be completed in the future.

Focus on the tasks that are most essential first before shifting to more essential assignments. It ensures you're progressing with the tasks important to you, and will help you stay away from getting caught up in lesser important activities.

Assigning tasks and working With Others

Another crucial aspect of managing your time is the ability to delegate work and effectively work with other people. If you're pressed for time It can be tempting to attempt to handle everything by yourself. But it's not the most effective or efficient strategy.

In order to effectively delegate work to your employees, follow these tips:

Determine tasks that are best assigned to other people. It could be tasks which are not within your expertise, or work that could be done more efficiently by an individual.

Pick the appropriate individual for the job, depending on their expertise and their availability. Take note of who in your group could be the best fit for the task and also whether they're able to commit sufficient time and resources to accomplish the task.

Be clear about what has to be accomplished and the deadlines or requirements. When you delegate jobs, you need to clearly define the information you require and when you'll need it. Be sure that the person delegating your task is aware of the job and is equipped with the knowledge required to finish it efficiently.

Give support and assistance in order to make sure you're able to complete the job with ease. If you're delegating the job you must be accessible to assist with questions and give guidance when required. This can ensure the job is done correctly and in accordance with your expectations.

Apart from delegating work It is also essential to be able to communicate effectively with colleagues. This could involve working in projects, soliciting input and feedback and forming good relationships with your colleagues. When you work well with other people it is possible to achieve more performance and efficiency on your job, and also build a strong community of peers and mentors.

Instruments to Manage Your Time during the 80-hour Week. Week

The demands of a full 80-hour week may be difficult However, it doesn't have to seem difficult. Through implementing efficient methods for managing time and using appropriate equipment and tools that will help you stay organised efficiently, productive, and productive in the midst of challenging work hours. Utilizing the best tools and resources is able to assist you in managing your time in a busy 80-hour workweek. There are several tools you could use to assist you in managing your time in a more efficient manner.

Time-Tracking Apps

Time-tracking applications are a great instrument to manage your time throughout a lengthy working week. Applications such as Toggl, RescueTime, and Harvest let you track your time spent on various projects and tasks, which allows you to see what you're doing and adjust as necessary. They can also assist to prioritize your tasks to ensure you're on the right track towards your objectives.

Project Management Tools

Tools for managing projects such as Asana, Trello, and Basecamp can be useful to organize your work time the long working week. They let you manage your tasks by task and project as well as assigning deadlines and responsibilities and work with colleagues. With the help of project management software help you keep track of your workload and be sure that you're achieving your deadlines and reaching your objectives.

Calendar Apps

Calendar software such as Google Calendar, Outlook, and Apple Calendar can be invaluable to manage your time throughout the long working week. They let you organize appointments, meetings and deadlines. They also allow you to schedule reminders and messages to help you stay on the right schedule. If you use a calendar app it will help you ensure you're effectively managing your time and getting the most out of your working week.

Automation Tools

Automated tools such as IFTTT Zapier, IFTTT, or Automate.io are also useful to organize your time throughout the long hours of work. They let you automate the repetitive routines, including sending out emails and scheduling posts on social media as well as organizing your documents. With these tools to automate your work, you'll reduce time, and also free time to focus on more pressing jobs.

Focus Apps

The apps for focus such as Forest, StayFocusd, and Freedom are useful for keeping track of your time and stay concentrated throughout a busy working week. These applications can help you avoid the distractions of apps and websites and set timers for breaks and working hours as well as track your performance. With focus apps, you will be able to stay away from distractions while focusing on work when you are working for a long time.

The management of your time in an working week of 80 hours isn't easy, but when you use the appropriate equipment and tools, it is possible to remain productive, organized and productive. Tools for tracking time as well as project management tools scheduling tools, automatization software and focus apps could prove useful in controlling your time and reaching the goals you set. If you're putting in an 8-hour week take a look at incorporating the tools listed above into your schedule to help remain on the right track to achieve the success you want. If you have the proper equipment and tools to help you succeed, you'll be able to handle even the toughest week-long work schedules.

A well-organized time management system is vital in surviving the stressful 80 hour Work Week. Through prioritizing your work and delegating tasks when necessary and being able to work effectively in collaboration with other people, you'll be able to maximize your time, and increase performance and effectiveness. In the subsequent sections, we'll look at some more strategies and methods for tackling the pressures that come with the Work Week and achieving your career goals.

Chapter 3: Managing Your Energy

Mincreasing your productivity is essential in surviving the Work Week, but it's not the only thing to take into consideration. It's equally important to manage your daily energy levels to ensure that you keep your focus, focused, and energized. In this section we'll look at some of the practical ways to manage your energy level and making the most of your day to work.

Understanding Your Energy Levels

To be able to effectively regulate your energy you must understand the way your energy levels change during the day. The majority of people experience natural highs and lows in their energy levels throughout the day. This is commonly referred to as "circadian rhythms". The rhythms of these cycles are affected by a variety of factors, including your eating habits, sleep schedule or exercise regimen which can differ between individuals.

For a better understanding of your personal cycle of rhythms in the night, you can track your energy levels over a week. Note when you feel the most focus and alert, as well as the times when you feel fatigued or distracted. This could help you determine patterns and modify your timetable accordingly.

Strategies for Managing Your Energy

When you know the state of your energy levels, then you'll be able to start implementing strategies to control your energy levels throughout your entire day. The most effective methods are:

Take regular breaks: Taking breaks throughout your day will keep you active and focus. Consider taking a stroll in the morning, stretching, or breathing deeply.

Experimenting outside: Being exposed to sunlight and fresh air can increase the energy level of your body and boost your mood. Consider taking a walk on your lunch break or even scheduling meetings outdoors as often as you can.

Eat for energy The food you eat plays an important impact on your energy levels throughout your day. In order to stay energetic, you should focus on eating a healthy, balanced food plan with lots of fresh food items, protein that is lean, as well as nutritious fats.

Drinking enough water: dehydration will reduce your energy levels and make you feel tired and distracted. Be sure to drink lots of fluids throughout your day. You may also want to consider adding electrolytes-rich drinks like coconut water, or beverages for sports to your diet.

Prioritizing your sleep: Getting sufficient sleep is essential for maintaining your performance levels. You should aim for around 7 to 8 hours of rest each at night. Establish regular sleep schedules for regulating your cycle of sleep.

Creating a Productive Environment

As well as controlling your energy level It is also essential to ensure a conducive work environment in order to reduce energy consumption. It can be as simple as:

Avoiding distractions such as email notifications, social media, as well as noisy colleagues can drain of your energy. You might want to consider using noise-cancelling headphones, blocking websites that distract you or even planning "focus time" when you have uninterrupted work.

Improve your workspace Your workspace's physical layout can influence your energy levels. You should ensure that your space is bright and comfortable think about adding ergonomic devices including a stand-up desk or an ergonomic chairs.

Align your work based on the energy level: align your tasks in accordance with your energy level in order to finish important and urgent work during peak energy.

Personalizing your surroundings Then, think about making your space more personal to your personal preferences and requirements.

It could involve the addition of artwork or plants as well as playing some music or using essential oils for a relaxing atmosphere.

Tools To manage your energy levels Managing your level of energy is a crucial element of maintaining efficiency and concentration throughout your entire day. It can be difficult to figure out which direction to take in the process of getting your energy levels up. There are, fortunately, numerous instruments and resources to help you control your energy levels and remain efficient. Below are a few tools you should take into consideration:

Sleep trackers getting enough rest is vital to keep your energy levels all day. Sleep tracking applications such as Sleep Cycle, Pillow, and SleepScore are able to help keep track of your sleeping patterns, evaluate the level of sleep you get, and offer suggestions for improving your sleeping habits.

Apps for meditation: Doing meditation can be a wonderful way to lower stress and improve the level of energy. Applications like

Headspace, Calm, and Insight Timer offer guided meditations along with other mindful exercises which can allow you to relax and refresh.

*Time management applications poor time management could result in fatigue and burnout. Tools for managing your time like Trello, Asana, and RescueTime are able to help you prioritize activities, organize your schedule to avoid overloading yourself.

Apps for fitness: Exercising is a crucial aspect of keeping energy levels high and maintaining general well-being. Fitness apps such as Nike Training Club, Fitbit and MyFitnessPal allow you to track your exercise routine, establish objectives, and keep track of your performance.

Blue filtering of light: Exposed to blue light from electronics may disrupt your natural sleep/wake cycle, and adversely impact the energy levels of your body. Blue light filters such as F.lux, Iris, and Twilight will help to decrease exposure to blue lights and increase sleeping quality.

Desk organizers: Unorganized workspaces are a source of distraction and exhaustion. Desk organizers such as the SimpleHouseware Desk Organizer, the Bamboo Desk Organizer, and the Mind Reader Desk Organizer can aid in keeping your space tidy and neat which reduces stress and increases efficiency.

When you incorporate these resources and tools to your everyday routine, it will help you increase the quality of your life and increase efficiency throughout your entire day. Try different tools and methods to determine the one that works for you. And don't hesitate to seek advice or assistance from others in case you are needing assistance. By using the appropriate techniques and mindset it is possible to control your energy levels, and meet your goals. By knowing your personal pattern of energy, and using successful strategies to control your energy levels throughout the day to stay on track efficient, productive, and motivated. In the next chapters, we'll examine some more strategies and methods for tackling the demands of an 80-hour Work Week and achieving your professional objectives.

Chapter 4: Maintaining Your Health And Well-Being

Working long hours could cause a lot of harm to your overall health and wellbeing physically as well as mentally. To be able to enjoy the time-consuming 80-hour Work Week, it's essential to put your health first and care for you both at and outside from work. In this section we'll look at some of the practical methods to ensure your well-being and health during the long hours of work.

Physical Health Strategies

If you're working for long periods of time, it's simple to forget about your physical wellbeing. Yet, making a priority of your health and fitness can keep you energized, engaged, and flexible. The most effective strategies for physical fitness comprise:

Being active and regular exercises can increase your energy levels, boost your mood, and lessen anxiety. A short stroll or stretching session can make huge impact.

Take breaks in between breaks: Alongside taking breaks to regulate your level of energy, regularly scheduled breaks throughout your day will also allow you to ensure your health. Make sure to get up and walk throughout the day every hour or two while also stretching while at work.

Healthy eating An energizing diet will aid in fueling your body and your brain to perform extended hours at working. Concentrate on eating whole food as well as lean proteins and lots of vegetables and fruits to provide your body with the nutrition it requires.

Manage stress: Having high levels of stress may affect the health of your body. You should consider incorporating techniques for managing stress like mindfulness, deep breathing or pilates in your daily routine.

Mental Health Strategies

Apart from physical health, it's crucial to pay attention to your mental well-being in the midst of an 80-hour Work Week. The long hours, the deadlines and high levels stress all can impact your mental wellbeing. A few effective ways to improve your mental health comprise:

Set boundaries: It's essential to establish boundaries for the personal and work life in order to prevent burnout. It could mean setting certain working hours, or carving out the time for leisure and hobbies.

Needing help Be open to ask for help from friends, colleagues or your family members when you're struggling. A supportive community can assist you in navigating the challenges that come with the hours Work Week.

Doing things for yourself such as bathing, studying a book or having massages can assist you in relaxing and recharging in the midst of long hours at work.

Creating a Supportive Work Environment

Also, creating a welcoming working environment could be a major factor in keeping you healthy and in good health through the long hours of your Work Week. A few effective ways to create an environment that is supportive of your work comprise:

Establishing relationships with your colleagues: A strong relationship with colleagues can make for a more positive and supportive workplace. Make the effort to get familiar with your colleagues and develop meaningful connections with them.

Communication with your boss If you're having trouble managing the long working hours, talk freely with your supervisor concerning your concerns. They might be able to offer support or suggestions for managing your work load.

Flexible work Try to incorporate flexibility into your timetable. This could involve doing some work at home or altering your schedule to meet other obligations.

Being healthy and in good health is essential to survive the long hours of Work Week. If you prioritize the health of your body and mind by creating a healthy workplace, and gaining your flexibility, you'll be able to be successful during your long working hours and meet your professional objectives.

BUILDING STRONG RELATIONSHIPS WITH CO-WORKERS

Eaffective communication is crucial to a successful workplace and especially when working long hours. Uncertainty, confusion and miscommunications can result in tension and anger. In this article we'll discuss some effective methods for effectively communicating during the eight-hour Work Week.

Clarifying Expectations

One of the key elements of a successful communication strategy is clearly defining expectations. If everyone is on the same page, it's simpler to remain productive, organized and focused. A few effective ways to define expectations are:

Setting specific objectives and deadlines: Make sure that your entire team knows what they're doing and the date they'll need to finish it.

Outlining the duties and roles: Be sure you know who's accountable for which tasks and make sure everyone is aware of the tasks they're responsible for.

Regularly communicating progress Updates on progress regularly helps everyone stay on course and avoid any surprise.

Managing Conflict

Conflict is a significant cause of frustration and stress throughout the long Work Week. But, with the right methods of communication, it is possible to handle conflict and solve conflicts in a positive way. The most effective strategies to manage conflict comprise:

Addressing problems early Do not wait until the situation has gotten out of control before addressing the issue. Make sure to address issues immediately when they are apparent in order to stop them from getting worse.

Active Listening: Pay attention attentively to the other person's viewpoint and attempt to comprehend their perspective.

Find common ground: Find areas where there is agreement and then work towards the most mutually beneficial solution.

Maintaining professional conduct In even the most heated of situations it is essential to keep an appropriate professional appearance and stay clear of personal assaults.

Collaboration Strategies

Collaboration is crucial to successful work However, it can be complicated when employees are at work for long periods of time. Effective collaboration methods comprise:

1. Set up communication channels that are clear Everyone should know how to talk with

one with one another, regardless of whether by phone, email or even instant messages.

2. Schedule regular check-ins. Regular checks-ins help keep everyone on the same page, and work effectively.

3. Utilizing collaboration tools such as Tools for collaboration such as Trello, Asana, and Slack aid in streamlined communications and help make collaboration easier.

4. Engaging in brainstorming and brainstorming sessions are a great way to generate fresh ways of approaching challenges and concepts.

SELF-CARE STRATEGIES

Self-care is essential to survive the long hours of Work Week. This can assist you in staying healthy, focused and enthusiastic throughout the long work hours. In this article we'll discuss some effective self-care methods to help maintain your health in and out of the workplace.

Mindfulness Techniques

Techniques for mindfulness like meditation, deep breathing, as well as pilates all can help to reduce stress and help improve concentration. The most effective strategies for mindfulness include:

Regular breaks are a good way to concentrate on your breathing or meditate.

Engaging in pilates, or any other exercises to ease tension and ease anxiety.

Relaxing with soothing music or sound to aid in the state of relaxation.

Engaging in activities of creativity like drawing, painting or writing, can help to calm your mind.

Mindfulness-based tools allow you to remain present and mindful of your feelings, thoughts and emotions with no judgment. They help to lower anxiety and stress, boost concentration and focus, and enhance overall wellbeing. It isn't easy to integrate mindfulness practices into your everyday routine. However you can find a range of resources and tools available that will help you to practice mindfulness. These are a few tools you should think about:

The apps for Meditation: Meditation can be an excellent way to develop mindfulness. Apps such as Headspace, Calm, and Insight Timer offer guided meditations along with other mindful exercises which can assist you in relaxing and keep your mind in the present.

Mindfulness journals: Recording your thoughts and feelings will aid in becoming conscious of them, and to take them into consideration in a calm method. Mindfulness journals such as The Five Minute Journal, The Happiness Planner, and The Mindfulness Journal offer prompts and activities that will aid you in developing a mindfulness habit.

Breathing exercises: focusing on your breathing is an easy and efficient technique to cultivate mindfulness. Apps such as Breathe2Relax, Breathing Zone, and

Pranayama provide breathing exercises as well as visualizations to assist you in relaxing and remaining in the present.

Journals for gratitude: The practice of practicing gratitude is a great way to develop an optimistic mindset, and help reduce stress. Gratitude journals such as The Gratitude Journal for Women, The Five Minute Journal and The Happiness Planner offer prompts and activities that will aid you in developing an appreciation practice.

Mindfulness bells: Mindfulness alarms are sound cues that keep you focused all day long. Applications like Mindbell, ZenAlarm, and Mindful Clock offer customizable mindfulness bells to assist you to remain conscious throughout your day.

When you incorporate these resources and tools in your routine, it is possible to enhance your meditation practice, and benefit from decreased stress, better concentration, and better overall well-being. Try different methods and strategies to discover which one works for you. And don't hesitate to seek assistance or advice from other people in case you are struggling. By using the appropriate methods and mindset it is possible to develop an effective mindfulness routine and enhance your overall wellbeing.

Social Support Strategies

A strong community of support can prove extremely helpful during the Work Week. The most effective strategies for social support comprise:

Establishing relationships with coworkers for a more supportive working environment.

Making contact with loved ones and friends in the off-hours to keep an equilibrium between life and work.

Participating in professional associations or online forums to network with people in your industry.

A counsellor or therapist if you need it.

Resources For Building A Professional Network:

1. LinkedIn: LinkedIn is a well-known professional social network which allows users to set up an account, network to colleagues and leaders in the industry and join groups that are relevant to them, as well as engage in information that's relevant to their industry. It's a great device for establishing and growing your professional networks It also offers multiple opportunities for networking as well as learning as well as job-searching.

2. Industry events: Going to trade shows, workshops, conferences and meetings can be a great means to network with other professionals within your industry, get advice from the experts and uncover exciting job openings. Examples of events in the industry are those like the Consumer Electronics Show (CES) and The Mobile World Congress (MWC) and the RSA Conference.

3. Professional associations: Getting involved in a professional organization that relates to your area of expertise can give you the ability to access resources, education and networking possibilities. Examples of professional associations are those like the Association for Computing Machinery (ACM) as well as the Institute of Electrical and Electronics Engineers (IEEE) as well as the International Association of Computer Science and Information Technology (IACSIT).

4. Online communities: Joining online communities like discussions boards, forums, as well as social media communities is a fantastic method of connecting with other people with similar interests and objectives. Some examples of online communities include Reddit's /r/ITCareerQuestions, Stack Overflow, and the DevOps Community.

5. Mentors and coaches: Establishing connections with coaches and mentors is a great means of getting assistance and advice from skilled experts. A few resources to find

coaches and mentors are SCORE an organization that is non-profit which provides no-cost mentoring and coaching to small and mid-sized business owners as well as entrepreneurs as well as the International Coach Federation (ICF) which is a professional association to coach coaches.

6. Alumni networks: Being connected to alumni of your college or university is an excellent resource to build your professional networking. There are many universities that have alumni associations and activities that offer opportunities to meet with people that share the same educational background and professional interests.

7. Volunteer groups: Volunteering with groups that relate to your profession or areas of interest is beneficial in terms of building your connections while also contributing to your community. A few examples of volunteer-based organizations are Code for America, a non-profit that connects technologists with community projects and

NetSquared is a worldwide community which supports the application of technology for positive social impact.

8. Meetup groups The Meetup platform that allows in-person gatherings as well as events for those with similar passions. There are a variety of meetup groups with a focus on IT-related and tech-related issues, like developing software, coding as well as cybersecurity.

9. Workshops and conferences: the event of attending events in industry and workshops, consider giving a talk or presentation at workshops or conferences. This will build your reputation as an authority in your field, and also give you opportunities to network with others in the field.

10. Events for networking Numerous cities hold gatherings specifically designed to professionals working within the medical, technology and IT fields. These networking events offer opportunities to connect with others from your area, share ideas and

experiences, as well as create new connections.

Through these sources as well as actively interacting with people within your industry You can create an effective and friendly professional network to aid you to achieve your goals and excel in a challenging workplace. Make sure you take networking seriously, with a positive outlook and always be open to opportunities and new views.

Conclusion

Communication is essential, as well as collaborating efficiently, and focusing on self-care is essential to survive the 80-hour Work Week. Through clarifying expectations, managing conflict and collaborating efficiently to stay focused and focused even through the long hours of work. Through self-care practices such as mindfulness, time management as well as social support to maintain the health of your body and mind all through the working week. In the concluding section, we'll look at other strategies to manage stress and maintaining your health throughout the 80-hour Work Week.

Chapter 5: Managing Stress and Burnout

Working long hours may cause excessive stress levels and burnout that can negatively impact the health of your employees, their well-being as well as your productivity. In this section we'll discuss some effective methods to reduce burning out and stress in the 80-hour Work Week.

Identifying Sources of Stress

The initial step towards managing burnout and stress is to identify sources of stress within your own personal life. Common sources of stress in the hours Work Week include:

The pressure of deadlines is high and the workload is heavy.

The long hours of work and the insufficient time for leisure and balance in work.

Problems with colleagues, supervisors, or other employees.

The pressure to exceed the expectations of others or perform at an elite performance.

The uncertainty or instabilities you face within your work or profession.

Imposter The illusion of your character

Stress can have a profound influence on your physical as well as mental wellbeing, and it is crucial to determine stress-related factors throughout your day so you can make measures to reduce and manage stress levels. It can be difficult to determine precisely what's driving the anxiety. Here are some methods to find the sources of stress in your lives:

Create a stress journal The use of a stress journal will help you keep track of the stress levels of your body and pinpoint patterns that you see in your routine. Every day, record the situations and incidents that made you stressed, along with your reaction to these events. This helps you pinpoint the stressors that are recurring and devise strategies to manage them.

Do a stress test You can find a range of assessments for stress available online which can assist you in identifying factors that cause stress in your daily life. They may inquire regarding your relationship, job as well as your financial position, among others that may cause stress.

Be aware of physical signs Stress may manifest in physical signs like muscular tension, headaches and stomach pain. Being aware of these signs could help you determine the root of tension. If, for instance, you are constantly suffering from headaches after being at work for long periods and you are stressed about your work, it may be an important source stress.

Review your timetable It is possible for your schedule to contribute to stress when it's too full or not well-balanced. Review your agenda and consider whether you're doing more than you can handle or ignoring essential self-care routines like exercising as well as rest.

Consider your core values: Stress is often caused by an inconsistency between your values and needs of your life. Spend some time reflecting on your core values and see how they are reflected in your work or relationships as well as other areas of your daily life.

Ask for feedback from people around you There are times when it can be hard to pinpoint the sources of stress in yourself or even discern when you're overwhelmed. Ask for feedback from your trusted relatives, friends or even colleagues who are familiar with you and could be able provide some view.

Finding the sources of stress in your daily life is the first step to controlling your stress and reducing its levels. With these methods and techniques, you'll be able to develop an understanding of the factors the cause of your stress and then implement steps to reduce the issue. Be gentle and understanding when you are working to decrease stress. And do not be afraid to seek help from a professional when you require it.

Developing Coping Strategies

The right strategies for managing stress can assist you in managing anxiety and avoid burnout throughout the gruelling 80-hour Work Week. The most effective strategies for managing stress are:

Practice mindfulness practices like meditation, deep breathing.

Participating in regular exercise helps reduce stress and improve the mood.

Engaging with family, friends or colleagues can help reduce the feeling of loneliness.

You can pursue hobbies, or any other activity that give you pleasure and peace.

Inquiring for professional assistance, such as therapy or counseling should you require it.

Managing Burnout

The term "burnout" refers to a condition of mental, emotional physical, and mental exhaustion which may be caused by prolonged stress. If it is not managed, the effects of burnout may have adverse effects on the health of your body and overall well-being.

Burnout can be described as a form of stress caused by work which can be very serious for both mental and physical effects on your health. It is in the event that you feel exhausted physically and emotionally exhausted, as well as not able to cope with the requirements of your job. These are the most common signs of burnout at work:

The feeling of being emotionally tired, drained or depleted can be a indicator of burnout. There is a feeling that you've got nothing to contribute and you've lost interest in the work you do.

The term "depersonalization" refers to the feeling of cynicism or detachment toward your work, coworkers and clients. There is a feeling that you're doing your thing and don't feel empathy for others.

A decrease in performance may affect your ability do your job efficiently. It is possible that you have trouble focusing on your decisions or working on tasks within the timeframe.

Physical signs: Burnout may cause physical manifestations like headaches, muscle tension and stomach problems. The symptoms could indicate your body is experiencing severe pressure.

Sleep disturbances and burnout: This can impact your sleep and cause insomnia, or trouble getting or staying asleep.

The loss of enthusiasm A lack of interest can lead your interest to wane at work, or in other pursuits you used to take pleasure in. There may be a feeling of a lack of motivation, and you may experience difficulty getting pleasure from your activities.

An increase in irritability can result in you feeling angry or even angry more frequently. It is possible to snap at your loved ones or colleagues on minor matters.

A decrease in satisfaction can result in a decrease of contentment with work and your life. There is a feeling that you're trapped in your routine and you've lost focus on the goals you have set and your values.

Effective strategies to deal with burning out include:

Set up healthy work limits and recognizing the need to say"no" when it is necessary.

It is important to prioritize self-care such as exercising as well as meditation and restorative activities.

Recognizing and challenging negative thinking or attitudes that lead to burning out.

It is important to have time off at work in order for rest and recharging whenever you need to.

Consider seeking professional assistance if signs are present.

If you're exhibiting signs of stress, you need that you take action to reduce the issue of burnout. You could talk to your boss about changing the work load or getting advice from a therapist or counselor. Keep in mind that burning out is a major issue which requires care and attention. If you take steps to reduce your stress levels and focus on your health, you will overcome burnout and restore enthusiasm for job.

Building Resilience to adjust and bounce back from adversity and stress. Being resilient can allow you to succeed during your 80-hour Work Week and maintain your overall health and wellbeing. The most effective ways to build resilience are:

Establishing solid relationships between friends, colleagues and loved ones.

A feeling of meaning and purpose within your personal and professional your life.

Concentrate on the positive aspects of your existence.

Finding opportunities for growth and growth.

Keep a spirit of humor and a sense of perspective.

Chapter 6: Achieving Success during the 80 Hour Work Week

Long working hours can be difficult, however they could also provide opportunities for development and growth. In this section we'll discuss some effective methods to achieve success in the 80-hour Work Week.

Goal Setting

Setting goals that are effective is essential to success in the hours Work Week. When you establish clear, precise objectives, you will be engaged and focus even through lengthy work hours or moments of high stress. The goal setting process gives you a sense of satisfaction and optimism will help you get throughout the week. A few effective methods for goal making comprise:

The goal setting process should be specific and measurable in line with your ideals and goals.

Condensing bigger goals into smaller, manageable task.

Set deadlines and set milestones to monitor the progress.

Recognizing achievements as they happen to keep you motivated.

Effective Goal Setting Tools And Frameworks

Utilizing tools to set goals specifically and frameworks is an effective method to set clear, concrete goals, and to work towards the goals. Below are a few instruments and frameworks of a popular nature which can assist you in creating and setting clear achievable goals that are measurable:

SMART Goals: SMART Goals is an extremely popular framework for setting goals which means Specific, Measurable and Achievable time-bound and relevant. This tool will assist you in creating precise and measurable objectives that target the desired outcome.

OKR is the acronym as Objectives and Key Results. This framework is employed by a variety of successful businesses for helping align personal goals and those of teams with larger goals of the organization. The tool focuses on setting challenging and achievable goals that are specific and have an underlying goal.

GROW Model: GROW stands for Goal and Reality. It also stands for Options and will. The GROW model is commonly utilized in coaching and mentorship for helping individuals establish and reach their targets. The GROW model stresses the necessity of understanding your present circumstances and exploring a variety of ways to reach your goals.

Eisenhower Matrix: The Eisenhower Matrix is a tool for productivity that helps you to prioritize your goals according to their importance and urgency. It is broken down in four areas: important, significant, however not urgent essential but not urgent but not important or urgent, and neither urgent nor significant nor urgent.

Habitica: Habitica is a game-based productivity application that will assist you in setting and achieving goals by transforming your to-do lists into games. Habitica rewards users with points for accomplishing tasks and helping you build healthy habits, which makes goal-setting easier and more enjoyable.

Trello It is a task management tool that helps to break large goals into more manageable projects. Trello makes use of a visual boards and cards that assist you with organizing the goals you want to achieve and keep track of the progress you make.

A 90-Day Calendar: A 90-Day planner is a goal-setting tool which is focused on setting and reaching targets within a 90-day timeframe. It emphasizes that it is important to set realistic but challenging goals, and breaks them into small, manageable steps.

Pomodoro Technique: The Pomodoro Technique can be a time-management device that helps to stay on track and be productive in achieving your objectives. This technique involves breaking down your day into 25 minute intervals that are followed by a quick break and continuing the sequence.

Vision Board A vision board can be described as an image representation of your objectives and hopes. It is made up of pictures, text, or other elements of visual design that can are motivating and inspiring. It serves as a continuous visual reminder of your goal and will help you stay in the right direction and on track.

Mind Mapping Mind mapping is an effective tool for brainstorming that will aid you in organizing your ideas and thoughts. It involves making an image of your objectives and the steps required to reach the goals. Mind mapping helps to see the bigger idea and reduce complex objectives into simpler actions.

Habit Tracker The habit tracker is an application that will help to establish and monitor positive behaviors. This tool is used to create your list of behaviors that you wish to develop as well as tracking your improvement throughout the course of time. The habit tracker can assist you to remain accountable and keep you inspired to reach the goals you set for yourself.

A good accountability buddy An accountability partner can aid in keeping you on track and accountable for your objectives. The method involves locating someone who is working towards the same goals as you and keeping in touch often to keep track of your progress and give assistance.

Utilizing these tools for setting goals and methods can help you establish and meet your goals faster. You may be looking to create healthy habits, prioritize your goals or align goals with larger organizational objectives, there's a solution on the market that will aid you to achieve your goals.

Staying Motivated

Maintaining motivation throughout the hours of Work Week can be challenging However, it's crucial to getting to your goals, progressing in achieving your goals. A few effective ways to stay inspired are:

1. Concentrating on your mission and the values you hold to remain active and motivated.

2. Recognizing small victories as you go to keep the momentum.

3. Inquiring for feedback and help from your supervisors and colleagues in order in order to stay focused.

4. Be positive and hopeful, even in difficult circumstances.

5. Do yourself a favor every now and then!

Tools To Help You Stay Motivated:

Quotes from inspirational authors websites like BrainyQuote or Goodreads have a variety of motivational quotations. It is also possible to follow the accounts of motivational people on social media including Instagram and Twitter.

Podcasts for motivation: The most popular inspirational podcasts are The Tony Robbins Show, The Brendon Show as well as The Daily Boost.

Vision boards Create your own vision board with the cork board or poster board. Or, you can use digital platforms such as Canva and Pinterest.

"Affirmations": Applications such ThinkUp, I Am and Headspace provide a range of affirmations which are customizable and you can hear every day.

Daily planners: Applications such as Todoist, Trello or Asana are able to help you handle your day-to-day tasks and keep well-organized.

Accountability Partner Find accountability partners through Facebook or on apps such as Focusmate as well as Coach.me.

"Motivational" books: Top selling motivational titles are "The 7 Habits of Highly Effective People" written by Stephen Covey

"Atomic Habits" by James Clear, and "The Power of Positive Thinking" written by Norman Vincent Peale.

Motivational videos on YouTube channels such as TED, Goalcast and Be Inspired have a broad selection of motivational video.

Meditation applications: Some popular meditation applications include Headspace, Calm and Insight Timer.

Gratitude journal: Apps such as Gratitude and Happyfeed permit users to make your own daily gratitude journal, and keep track of the progress you make.

Continuing Education and Professional Development

Additionally, continuous training and development for professionals could be a powerful method to be successful in the 80-hour Work Week.

Continuous education and professional growth can prove to be a powerful method to be successful during working for 80 hours by a variety of ways:

Current knowledge and abilities Professional training can keep you updated on the most recent advancements and trends in your area. It will help you remain current and relevant, as well as improve your worth in the role of an employer.

Enhance your job performance and productivity professional development may assist you in improving your job performance, by providing you with the knowledge and skills that you require to succeed in your job. This will make you more effective and efficient at your job as well as increase your odds of being successful.

Professional advancement: Continued learning and professional development will assist you in preparing for job advancement opportunities like promotions, or even the possibility of a new job. It can assist you in achieving your professional goals and rise upwards in your career.

Personal development: Professional growth helps you develop personally, by increasing your self-confidence as well as expanding your knowledge while also improving your communication skills and leadership capabilities.

Opportunities to network Opportunities for continuing education and professional growth events offer the opportunity to network and meet others working in your area. These events can assist you in establishing connections and broaden your professional circle that can result in possibilities for collaboration and opportunities.

Effective strategies to continue training and development for professionals include:

The pursuit of higher degrees or certificates within the field you are interested in.

Attending conferences or seminars to keep up-to-date with the latest trends in the industry and top techniques.

Looking for advice or mentorship from more skilled colleagues.

Regular self-reflection and evaluation to determine the areas that need improvement and growth.

Websites and resources can aid in continuing education while you are working an hour week

Coursera: Coursera is an online platform for learning that provides classes and specializations offered by leading universities and colleges all over the world. It provides a broad range of classes in the fields of technology as well as business and other areas, many of which are self-paced, and may be completed according to your personal timetable.

Udemy: Udemy is another famous online learning platform that provides courses in a range of topics including IT and tech. The majority of its classes are self-paced so learners can take courses at their personal pace according to your timing.

Lynda.com: Lynda.com is an online platform for learning that provides classes in technology, business as well as other areas. It has a broad selection of classes that are led by professionals in the field and allows you to learn according to your own time.

Codecademy: Codecademy is an online platform for learning and training that specialises in teaching programming and coding abilities. It provides interactive lessons as well as tutorials to assist you in learning new techniques and keep up-to-date on the most recent technological trends.

LinkedIn Learning LinkedIn Learning can be described as a professional-oriented platform offering various lessons and training on subjects including technology, leadership, as well as managing projects. There are courses that are taught by professionals in the field who can help you study at your own speed at your own time.

Udacity: Udacity is an online learning platform which offers classes and nanodegrees in science, the fields of business, technology as well as other areas. They offer self-paced, self-paced learning that you can complete on your own timetable and also mentoring and career assistance to assist you in achieving your goals.

Khan Academy: Khan Academy is a non-profit institution which offers online classes as well as tutorials for a wide range of subjects like sciences, math as well as computer programming. They offer self-paced, interactive courses which can be taken at your own pace, and is an excellent tool for revising basics and understanding new ideas.

Skillshare: Skillshare is an online platform to learn that gives classes in business, design technologies, design, and many different fields. Courses are that are taught by experts from the industry, and allows you to learn in your own way and on your own time.

All in all, ongoing training and development for professionals could be an investment for your professional as well as personal development, particularly during long working periods. If you keep up to date with the most recent trends within your field, enhancing the performance of your employees, as well as increasing your networks to boost your chances to succeed and meet your goals in career.

Conclusion

To be successful during the hours Work Week requires effective goal planning, managing time and motivation. It also requires support and continuous professional growth. With clear objectives and focusing your time efficiently while remaining motivated, creating an effective support system, and seeking out ongoing training and growth to ensure you are thriving during working long hours and accomplish your professional objectives. In this final section, we'll go over the key lessons learned and provide some thoughts about how to survive and succeeding in the hours of the Work Week.

Achieving your goals during the eight-hour Week: Week:

The eight-hour Work Week can be challenging However, it can offer opportunities for development and growth. Through defining expectations as well as managing conflict, working on self-care and creating strategies to succeed to thrive in working long hours and meet your goals in the workplace.

In this book we've discussed effective strategies for managing and succeeding in the hours Work Week. We've talked about the importance of efficient communication, collaboration as well as self-care. We've given concrete strategies and tools for managing stress, gaining resilient, and reaching successful outcomes.

A few of the most significant takeaways from this book are:

Set clear expectations with your colleagues, supervisors, and customers to avoid confusion and uncertainty.

Effectively manage conflict by staying in a calm state, paying attention and pursuing win-win solutions.

Utilize self-care strategies such as mindfulness, managing your time, and support from friends to keep your overall health and wellbeing.

Recognize the causes of stress, create strategies for coping, and deal with the effects of burnout efficiently.

Create clear and specific objectives, plan your time effectively and remain focused to attain your goals during the eight hours of Work Week.

Create a solid support system to continue your education and professional growth in addition to seeking advice and mentorship from colleagues who have more experience.

Resources for Additional Support and Guidance

The American Institute of Stress - The organization offers resources as well as support to those who suffer from burning out and stress. They also offer education materials including workshops, online classes on managing stress and resilience.

The National Alliance on Mental Illness (NAMI) is a non-profit organization that offers support and advocacy to those and their families affected mental disease. They provide resources and help groups for people suffering from anxiety, stress, or burning out.

The Society for Human Resource Management (SHRM) The Society for Human Resource Management (SHRM) gives support and resources to HR professionals as well as employees. They provide tools and information to help manage stress and encourage health and well-being at work.

The American Psychological Association (APA) is a resource organization that provides assistance as well as support to those who are suffering from anxiety, stress and burnout. They also provide advice on the mental health of people, self-care as well as professional growth.

It is the Work-Life Balance Institute - This company provides guidance and support those who want to find a balance between their lives at work and in private. They offer coaching, workshops as well as online resources to manage stress, maintaining connections, and attaining working-life balance.

The Employee Assistance Programs (EAPs) - Numerous employers provide EAPs with confidential counselling and assistance for family members and employees. EAPs can prove to be an invaluable tool for managing stress levels and burning out.

Always remember that seeking help and advice is an indication of confidence and not weak points. Do not be afraid to ask to someone for assistance if you're suffering from fatigue or stress during the eight-hour Work Week. If you have the proper equipment and tools that you have, you will be able to thrive in the long hours of work and reach your goals in the workplace.

Utilizing these methods and strategies using these strategies and techniques, as well as taking advantage of some of the resources available, you'll be able to be successful during the long hours of work and meet your professional objectives. It is possible to maintain your physical and mental health and build lasting friendships with friends and colleagues as well as make a significant contribution to your company and your community.

The hours of the 80-hour Work Week can be challenging however, it could also offer the chance for growth in development and accomplishment. If you take a proactive and methodical approach to work and focusing on your well-being, health as well as personal development, you'll be more successful during your the long hours of work and accomplish your goals as a professional. I appreciate your time reading this and I hope you have a great time in your quest to be successful throughout the 80-hour Work Week.

Chapter 7: Understanding the Effects of Burnout

Being someone who has been through burnout for the first time I am aware of how debilitating it is. Burnout can be described as a condition of physical, mental, and mental exhaustion triggered due to stress or over-stress. This can affect all aspects of your lifestyle, from interactions with others as well as your general health and wellbeing. However, what is the root cause of burning out, and why does the issue so common in highly sought-after work?

The phenomenon of burnout is complex which can be manifested in different ways for various people. A few of the most prevalent signs of burnout are chronic anxiety, insomnia, fatigue or anxiety as well as depression. It's crucial to understand that burnout isn't the identical to depression, even though both conditions may overlap.

There are many causes that could contribute to the process of burning out, which include:

A high workload: If you're working all day long while juggling several projects as well as juggling tight time frames, it's easy to feel exhausted and overwhelmed.

Lack of control If you're concerned that there's no control over your workplace or the work you're given it may be difficult to remain motivated and interested.

Poor fit for the job Your job may not match your beliefs, values or talents It can be difficult to locate meaning and the purpose behind your job.

A lack of support If you are feeling lonely or not supported by colleagues or supervisors, it could be difficult to cope with the stress and keep yourself focused.

In the event that it seems like you're not receiving fair treatment or unfairly, it could be due to harassing, discrimination, or any other form of discrimination It can be difficult to maintain a positive outlook and perspective.

Stressors in your personal life When dealing with problems with your personal life, such as relationships, financial strain or health problems this can cause the symptoms of burnout.

The physical effects of burnout are significant. impact on your health. Stress can cause an increase in the chance of developing heart illness, high blood pressure as well as other heart-related issues. Stress can also affect the immune system, causing people to be more vulnerable to illness and infections. Issues with digestion like acid reflux IBS, acid reflux, as well as stomach ulcers, are prevalent among burnout sufferers.

It doesn't only affect physical health, but it may cause a serious impact on a person's mental and emotional wellbeing. The most frequent mental effects associated with burnout are depression. It can lead to feelings of despair or despair. The anxiety is another frequent symptom which can trigger anxiety as well as panic, anxiety, and. The burnout condition can cause irritation or anger which can result in people with a feeling of being emotionally exhausted and disengaged. It is crucial to deal with the physical, emotional and psychological consequences of stress to avoid further adverse effects for overall health.

The most common cause of burnout is highly-demanding jobs due to a variety of reasons. The most sought-after jobs typically come with the highest levels of responsibility, tension, and responsibility. If you're always trying to meet deadlines that are tight and manage large projects and ensure a high standard of efficiency, it could become easy to be stressed and tired.

Jobs that are in high demand often involve some level of mental strain. When you're dealing with a demanding client, managing hard-working colleagues, or managing complicated office politics, these jobs can drain you emotionally. Additionally, jobs that are highly sought-after are associated with an environment of stress and exhaustion. A lot of high-stress positions reward workers for their long working periods of time, depriving themselves of personal time and placing work ahead of anything other priorities. It could create a culture that is one where burning out is accepted as well as expected.

It's not only experiencing fatigue or stress due to working. It's a condition that is characterized by emotional, physical and mental exhaustion which can make you feel completely exhausted both physically and mentally. It is usually the result of constant stress. It is manifested by a sense of cynicism disconnection, and the feeling that you are overwhelmed.

Burnout's physical symptoms may be very severe, resulting in insomnia, fatigue headaches and weak immunity. The psychological consequences can be just as detrimental and can cause feeling of depression, anxiety and feelings of despair. Burnout's psychological consequences can be equally devastating as the physical ones, including decreased satisfaction at work as well as a loss of motivation and an eroding feeling of satisfaction.

There's no wonder that the phenomenon of burnout occurs in a lot of high-demand job positions. There is a pressure to perform at an extremely very high standard, in conjunction with long working hours and a lack of time for self-care can easily result in exhaustion. Additionally that, the competitive demands of a lot of high-demand jobs may create a workplace which can be stressful and high-stressing.

Based on my personal experience I've felt burnout's effects first-hand. Being a long-time worker in balancing working a full-time job and the demands of my family and being constantly under need to work at an extremely high standard eventually wore me out. I was overwhelmed all the time and unable to concentrate and be productive in my work while also feeling was unable to enjoy the things that I had previously enjoyed.

The good thing is that burning out isn't unavoidable, and there are ways to avoid it, or even recover from it. In the subsequent sections, we'll explore various strategies which can assist you in recovering from burnout and reenergize your body and mind, even while you work in an occupation that is highly-demanding.

Chapter 8: Signs and Symptoms of Burnout

It can be difficult to tell when burnout is coming up for the person you are, and it's always simple to identify warning signs or symptoms while you're at the midst of it. In this article we'll discuss ways to identify burnout, different types of burnout and warning indicators to look for in you and other people.

If you're suffering from fatigue, you may appear as if you're going through your routine. It's possible to feel exhausted in your work, demotivated, or even unproductive. There's a chance your mood is more stressed in comparison to the norm, or it's difficult to focus. It's crucial to be aware of the signs of stress and act before it becomes overwhelming.

The best way to spot burnout is by paying the mental and physical condition. Do you feel more exhausted more than normal, even after a having a good night's rest? Are you struggling to fall asleep or sleeping? Are you stressed or annoyed for no motive? Are you having trouble focusing or recall certain things?

Another method to detect burnout is by paying attention to the way you work. Do you find yourself putting off work more often than you would like, or have difficulties launching projects? Do you make more errors than normal and struggling to make deadlines? Are you struggling to stay organised or managing your time efficiently?

It's not a quick fix it's a gradual process that could be months, or years to build. There are three phases of burnout: honeymoon that follows the peak of stress and the chronic burnout.

When you're in the honeymoon stage it is possible to feel euphoric and motivated by the work you've done. You may be working the long hours and working far, but you're loving what you're doing. But, it can cause the development of stress. You become overloaded and stressed. It is possible that you will struggle to sleep as well as you could be tempted to use harmful coping methods like drinking or using drugs to deal with the stress.

If you do not respond to the signs of stress, you could become chronically burned out. In this phase it is possible to feel emotional physical and mentally exhausted depressed and depressed. The possibility is that you begin to feel isolated from friends and family as well as feeling that your job doesn't really matter any more.

If you're feeling burnt out you need to get it addressed before the situation becomes overwhelming. There are a few indicators to look out for:

Physical signs like stomachaches, headaches or muscular tension

The emotional symptoms include an anxiety or irritability depression

Reduced productivity or performance at work

Refrain from working or other social events

Excessive use of drugs, alcohol, or food in order to manage the stress

Bedwetting or other sleep disruptions

Are you feeling that you don't have any control over your job or private life

You feel like you'ren't having an impact or you don't have a role to play?

All women over 40 need to be aware of burning out and perimenopausal symptoms can be similar symptoms that could make it difficult to differentiate between them.

The most common signs of burnout are physical and mental exhaustion, depression and cynicism, feelings that you are not doing enough or lacking satisfaction, as well as decreased productivity.

In the same way, typical symptoms of menopausal perimenopausal symptoms can also include physical manifestations like hot flashes, night sweats insomnia, and sleep disruptions and emotions such as anger as well as depression, anxiety and irritability. It is important to keep in mind that perimenopausal changes are an internal process that is affecting women who are approaching menopausal and burnout can be a outcome of continuous stress at work. If you're experiencing some of these symptoms you should consult with a medical professional in order to pinpoint the causes and seek out the proper medical treatment.

I believed I was sorted out, a successful job and beautiful kids. However, as time passed, the pressures of my job that was extremely stressful began taking their toll on me. I would work lengthy hours in working, and even when I came back home, I was connected to my mobile as well as my laptop. It was like I never really had the ability to unplug.

In the beginning, I thought that I was simply fatigued. As time passed I noticed different signs. I became angry and irritable in my relationship with my children as well as angry with my colleagues for without reason. I was struggling to sleep and was dependent ever more heavily on coffee for energy to go through the workday. I began to experience the dread of each Sunday night, realizing that my week was just about to begin. I noticed that I was losing enthusiasm for activities I enjoyed and began to avoid social occasions. I was feeling feelings of despair and despair, feeling as if I could not keep up in the demands of my work and life. That was when I realized that I was suffering from exhaustion.

I can remember sitting at a conference with my boss and trying to remain focused on the topic that was taking place. My mind was going elsewhere and I was struggling with in keeping track of the conversation. At that point I felt a surge of fatigue wash over me. I was unable to contain the tears that began to pour out within my eyes. I quickly walked away and headed to the bathroom. There, I cried to my death. I was completely overwhelmed, as if I could not cope with requirements of my work as well as my private life.

The moment came as an awakening moment for me. I recognized that I'd been pushing myself to the limit over a long period of time and I had to make adjustments to prevent burning out completely. This wasn't an easy task, however by bringing a well-balanced approach to professional and personal life I managed to come back from the effects of burnout, and develop an easier way to live and working.

In the event that you're currently reading this article it's likely that you've had something like this. Perhaps you're exhausted and overwhelmed. You feel like you're at the edge of becoming exhausted. Maybe you've already hit that threshold and are trying to deal with the emotional, physical psychological, and physical consequences of burning out.

Whatever the case, it's essential to be aware of the warning indicators and signs of burnout to take the necessary steps prior to it becoming unmanageable. The process of burning out doesn't occur over night, but it is common to see warning signs which appear prior to reaching the point of no return.

Chapter 9: The Consequences of Ignoring Burnout

In the beginning, it may seem to be just a short-term feeling of fatigue. If it is not addressed the condition can have grave effects on your health, work, and your personal life. The absence of burnout could have lasting negative effects that could last for years before being overcome.

I've experienced the repercussions of not addressing burnout earlier during my career. I was the project manager at an enormous firm. I was extremely passionate about the work I did and determined to be an important part of the team. But as time passed forward I realized that I realized that the demands on my work were excessive. I had to work long days, taking on greater responsibilities than I could manage, and even sacrificing my own time in order to make deadlines. I could tell I was exhausted, but I wasn't willing to acknowledge it. I thought that if I persevered, it were going to get better. But, it wasn't the scenario.

With time I began to feel how burnout affected my overall health. I felt constantly tired angry, stressed, and inability to focus. I was unable to fall asleep during the night and often awake feeling tired. Then I began to experience physical symptoms, like headaches and stomachaches. I was aware there was something wrong but I wasn't willing to leave work to deal with the issue. I was concerned that, should I do so it, I'd be viewed as weak and ineffective to meet the demands of my work.

However, I was not right. The fact that I ignored my burnout only increased the stress. I started to make errors at work, as well as miss important deadlines. My boss noticed and began to be more negative about my job. My coworkers began to leave me out, which made me feel more feeling lonely and isolated. I was so preoccupied with my work that I did not realise how much my life in general was in shambles. My marriage was in disarray and relations with my kids were in a state of tension. It wasn't until I had hit low that I understood the ramifications that I had ignored burnout.

The absence of burnout may have grave negative effects for your work, health as well as your personal life. Below are some typical negative long-term consequences of burnout

Physical health: Stress and fatigue can affect the health of your physical. The effects of chronic stress could lead to the development of high blood pressure as well as heart disease and various other issues with your heart. Additionally, it can affect the immunity, which makes people more susceptible to sickness as well as infections. The effects of burnout may also result in problems with digestion, such as acid reflux and irritable bowel syndrome as well as stomach ulcers.

Health: Mental stress could also have an important influence on your mental health. It may cause depression, despair and desperation. The result can be feeling of anxiety as well as panic, anxiety, and. The effects of burnout may cause irritation or anger. The result can be feeling emotional drained and disconnected. When it gets to a point, burning out may cause anxiety and depression issues.

Work: Neglecting burnout could negatively impact your professional career. The effects of burnout include low job satisfaction, lower efficiency, and failure to meet deadlines. Additionally, it can cause conflict with supervisors and coworkers. If not addressed, the issue of it could result in job losses or job changes.

Life outside of work: Burnout may impact your life in general. It could cause tension in friendships with friends and family. Additionally, it can cause a loss of interest in the things and hobbies that used to fill you with pleasure. The effects of burnout may cause feelings that you are disconnected and uninterested in your surroundings.

In spite of these dangers, many individuals continue to work hard and fail to recognize the symptoms of exhaustion. It is especially the case when working in highly-demanding jobs, as it is possible to be under pressure to be on the clock for long periods of time and adhere to tight deadlines. But, not addressing burnout could be an extremely risky game to be playing.

If not dealt with the burnout may get out of hand and become increasingly difficult to overcome. At some point, it could get out of control and require you to leave from work or leave your job altogether. When you act early it is possible to stay clear of these severe measures, and also recover of burnout prior to it gets to extreme.

Chapter 10: Strategies for Preventing Burnout

It can be hard to get over, but it's better to avoid burnout in the first place. In this article we'll discuss some ways to prevent burning out before it becomes a problem. The strategies are based on identifying the core values you hold dear, establishing safe boundaries, and handling your stress effectively.

The most crucial actions you can do in order to stop burnout is to establish the core values that define you. These are the beliefs and values which are the most important for you. Once you know the things that matter to you most and your family, you'll be able to make more informed decisions regarding how you spend your time and effort. It helps you concentrate only on things that are important and eliminate the ones that aren't.

For identifying your most important values, consider what is the most important for you in your the world. Common core values are the family, health, job as well as spiritual and individual growth. There are different values that are significant for you too. Note down your values and put them somewhere you are able to see them frequently. Being aware of your core values is crucial to avoid burning out. It will allow you to stay focussed on the things that matter most to you. It also forms the basis of your decision-making process. It will guide your decisions and behavior.

As an example, perhaps you think of your family as the most important value. This is then sustainability, as well as doing your best for the people as well as the planet. That means you are adamant about the time you spend with your beloved family members, but also think about the effect of your choices to the world and all those that surround you.

Once you have identified your primary values, you will be able to ensure that you align your professional and personal lives with these values. It can make to feel more satisfied as well as motivated and enthusiastic. This can also help you make decisions aligned with your beliefs which reduces the likelihood of being overwhelmed and burnt out.

To discover your most important beliefs, take some time to consider the things that matter to you most. Find out what causes you the greatest joy and happiness in your life and what is the reason you rise each day. You should also consider what are your absolutes that you can't compromise on when it comes to your life. When you are considering these ideals, make sure to be as precise as you can.

In the case of family, if it is one of the most important values for you, consider what exactly that means to you. Do you want to spend quality time with your family and friends and putting your kids' education first as well as personal development as well as creating a caring and peaceful home? Be specific with your beliefs will help you know what you really desire to put first in your the world and assist you in making decision-making and actions. It's crucial to recognize that the core values of everyone will appear different and that's fine. Most important is finding those values that are in alignment with the core of you and provide significance and meaning to your daily life.

Spend some time thinking about and then write down your top principles. When you've discovered the values, think about how they can be incorporated within your professional and personal daily life. This could involve setting boundaries by stating no to obligations which do not align with your beliefs Prioritizing your activities which align with the things that are the most important to you.

An additional method for avoiding burning out is to establish healthy limits. This includes knowing when you can not say "no" and knowing ways to guard your energy and time. When you create good boundaries, you're taking charge of your own life, and prioritizing your priorities.

For setting good boundaries, you must first start with identifying things that make you tired or create you to stress. These could include certain jobs or actions, certain individuals and circumstances. When you've determined these issues and made a strategy for the best way to handle these issues. It could mean delegating work or saying no to specific requests, or not allowing certain individuals or situations.

Work in corporate America can be stressful and stressful, often demanding endless hours of work, continuous communication as well as a never-ending work load. In this kind of setting it is often difficult to establish appropriate boundaries and to maintain the balance between work and life. There are a few reasons it can be difficult to set boundaries and a few practical suggestions for getting over those hurdles.

Fear of Consequences: A major reason that it may be difficult to define boundaries is anxiety of the consequences. Some employees worry that establishing limits can result in negative consequences like not being viewed as committed or not getting promotions.

The pressure to perform: Stress-inducing work environments often have stress-inducing environment which makes it challenging to prioritize your health. If employees are under need to be productive and be successful, they might compromise their own personal lives and health to avoid burning out.

The culture of overworking is prevalent. Many organizations have a culture of excessive work, with employees asked to work for long periods of time and answer work-related emails or messages during the normal hours of work. Within this type of culture it can be difficult. Establishing healthy boundaries in corporate America isn't easy since the culture stresses working all hours of the day and being accessible throughout the day. But, there are ways to define boundaries and focus on self-care within the workplace.

Another option is to think strategically about what and when you will communicate your limits. Instead of stating explicitly that you're unavailable, you can make important appointments outside of the work day and declare that you are currently engaged in an appointment. It is also possible to set certain time slots for tasks related to your job as well as make it clear that during those hours the time you are not answering calls or checking emails because of other obligations. My staff knows that I'll depart the office around 4.30PM everyday, and I'm off until 8.30PM at which point I'll get back in for a couple of hours to read emails. As I set specific boundaries for my time of availability but I'm mindful of the demands of a demand-driven culture of Corporate America. Through scheduling certain times to complete work and expressing the availability of my colleagues I'm able to take care of myself while remaining flexible to the needs of my work.

Another option is to engage in self-care in the workplace. Making short breaks during the day to stretch, reflect or even take an exercise session can help get your energy back and relieve stress but without affecting your efficiency. Also, make sure to prioritize tasks according to the importance of them and their urgency in order to concentrate on what is most important and delegate things that aren't as important and can be put off for.

If you're an executive in your organization, then you should also set healthy limits for your staff by focusing on work-life balance and urging others to follow suit. This could help to change the mindset of your company and help make it easier to prioritize self-care, which can aid in the retention of employees who are key to your business.

In the end, although it may be difficult to establish guidelines for healthy behavior in corporate America however, it's possible to focus on the self-care of employees and prevent burnout by using the right amount of creativity and strategic thinking.

It is important to be courteous and firm in establishing the boundaries. Make sure you are clear on your requirements but be considerate of others' expectations and needs. It is essential to begin by listing your top priorities and then focusing your attention on them prior to anything else. Make specific hours throughout the day to complete tasks that demand your full concentration and put them ahead of things that are less important. It is essential to avoid burning out and to maintain a healthy life-work equilibrium. This could include ensuring you get enough rest, following a balanced lifestyle, and engaging regularly in physical activity. A support network will help you keep the boundaries you set and help prevent burning out. These could include family members, friends, colleagues or family members who can appreciate the pressures of work and are able to provide emotional and moral support.

Set healthy boundaries when working in stressful work environments can be difficult yet it's essential in maintaining a healthy work/life balance, and also avoiding burning out. If you prioritize your work, establishing your boundaries, being assertive yet polite, focusing on self-care and establishing an environment of support to set and keep healthy boundaries within corporate America.

Also, managing stress efficiently can help prevent exhaustion. There are numerous strategies that you can implement to control stress. Some of them include exercises as well as meditation, deep breaths as well as relaxation methods. You must determine which will work best for your needs and then make it a routine aspect of your life.

One method that has been proven to be highly beneficial for dealing with anxiety is meditation. It involves keeping your focus in the present and getting rid of thoughts that distract you. Meditation regularly has been proven to lower anxiety and boost overall wellbeing.

I was taught the value of having healthy boundaries painfully. I was prone to saying"yes" to everything even if it meant that I had to compromise my own priorities and needs. I believed that working as a team member meant constantly putting other people first however, I soon realized that this could be the recipe for burnout. After months of all day and accepting requests from my coworkers and bosses I reached a point of no return. I felt exhausted, angry and always anxious. I recognized that I had to take a step back for me to prevent burnout.

The first step was choosing my values of the moment and making them a top priority. I came to realize that my family and health as well as my the development of my own self were most important to me over being constantly pleasing people. I also began to set boundaries in my life by kindly denying

111

demands that were not in alignment with my values. It wasn't an easy task initially however, I quickly realized that this was imperative for me to keep my overall health.

In the end, I tried mindfulness-based meditation to help to reduce anxiety. I discovered that this method allowed me to remain in a state of calm and focus when I was in stressful circumstances. Through focusing on the current moment I was able to let go of distractions thoughts and remain focused. Here are some instances of mindfulness exercises are available to try:

Meditation: Choose an area that is quiet and that you can relax for a short time. Relax your eyes and concentrate on the breath. Be aware of the feeling of air flowing in and out of your nose or the rising and falling in your chest. When your mind is wandering then gently draw your focus to the breath.

Body scan: Lay down on an yoga mat or a soft flooring. Take your eyes off and focus your focus to the physical sensations you feel within your body. Start with the high point of your head. You will move down the back to notice any spots of tension or pain. Once you're aware of any location, you can breathe deeply into it and work to let go of any tension.

Walking meditation: Locate an outdoor area that is quiet and that you can stroll in peace for a short time. Take a slow walk and be aware of the physical sensations you experience while walking. These include the feel of your feet rubbing against the floor or the motion in your hands. When your mind begins to wander, slowly bring your focus back to the physical sensations that accompany walking.

A mindful eating strategy: Select tiny pieces of food like an raisin, or a piece of chocolate. Take it into your palm take a close look at it taking note of the texture, shape as well as its hue. After that, slowly place it into your mouth. place it on your tongue with no chewing for at least a couple of minutes.

While you chew, be aware of the taste and feel of your mouth.

Meditation on loving-kindness: Relax in a quiet place and repeat in a quiet voice for your self: "May I be happy, may I be healthy, may I be safe, may I live with ease." In a short time think of someone you are concerned about and repeat the words to them. After that, spread the words for all living things.

Exercise can also be a fantastic way to decrease anxiety. The exercise process releases endorphins that will help increase your mood as well as reduce the anxiety and stress. Yoga can be a great way to lower stress levels and boost the general health and well-being of you. Yoga incorporates physical exercises together with deep breaths and meditation.

Time management that is effective can aid in reducing stress helping you prioritize your work and lessen the feeling of being overwhelmed. Chatting with family and friends members about stressors may aid in reducing anxiety and offer emotional assistance. Also, you can try out your hand at creative activities - participating in activities that stimulate creativity, such as writing, painting or even playing music, can assist to ease stress and increase the feeling of being well.

There are many strategies for managing stress. It's crucial to figure out the best method for you and then make stress-management regular in your daily routine.

Chapter 11: Strategies To Recover

Burnout is an issue that can be a major problem at work and could cause a myriad of detrimental consequences for both individuals as well as organizations. It is a condition of emotional, physical and mental exhaustion triggered by constant exposure to stress-inducing situations. It may trigger a range of symptoms like depression, anxiety, as well as physical ailments. If untreated, it may lead to severe physical and mental health concerns and could seriously affect individuals' ability to complete the job.

The good news is that recovery from burnout is achievable, and there are a variety of methods that people can employ to recover and manage burnout. One of the first steps to recovering from burnout is assessing the severity of your burning out. The assessment can help you identify the severity of your burnout, and help you create a recovery plan.

Another method to determine the severity of the severity of burnout is using an inventory of burnout. The inventory of burnout can be self-reported questionnaires which measure the intensity of symptoms associated with burnout. It is the Maslach Burnout Inventory is a commonly used inventory for burnout which evaluates three aspects of burnout: exhaustion emotionally as well as depersonalization and a decrease in satisfaction with life. The term "emotional exhaustion" refers to the feeling exhausted physically and emotionally. The term "depersonalization" refers to the feeling disconnection from the work environment as well as colleagues. A lower level of personal achievement indicates feeling less competent and success in the workplace.

The Maslach Burnout Inventory (MBI) is a tool for assessing copyrighted content which is why the MBI isn't typically accessible to the public for free. Important to know that interpreting and administering the MBI is a skill that requires special knowledge and training in the field of the field of mental health and burnout.

Another method to evaluate burnout is by using the self-assessment test. The questionnaires were intended to aid individuals in identifying symptoms of burnout, and evaluate the severity of their signs. Self-assessment tests are those from the Copenhagen Burnout Inventory and the Shirom Melamed Burnout Measure.

This is an example self-assessment of burnout questionnaires - take a moment to read every sentence and then rate the frequency you experience in this manner by using this scale.

0 = Never

1 = Very seldom (once or twice per year)

2. Sometimes (once or twice in a month)

3 = Usually (once or twice per week)

4 = Always (daily)

1. Physically and emotionally, I am tired and exhausted.

2. It's like I'm just doing nothing to improve my job or in my personal life.

3. I'm having difficulty sleeping or am experiencing sleep problems.

4. I'm frustrated, angry or irritable when I am with friends, colleagues or my family.

5. I'm feeling unappreciated and undervalued at work.

6. I have difficulty being able to stay focused or focus in my work.

7. I'm emotionally detuned or even numb.

8. I'm feeling a bit critical or cynical regarding my job or personal life.

9. I've lost interest and motivation for my work or my personal life.

10. I'm physically ill I am experiencing physical discomfort, like stomach or headaches.

Scoring:

You can add up the scores from each of the statements for a total score.

If your score is between 0 and 10, it implies that you're not suffering from burning out.

If the score of your overall ranges from 11-20, this could indicate that you're suffering from moderate burning out.

If your score ranges from 21-30, this implies that you're suffering from moderate burnout.

If the total score is higher than 31 this suggests you're suffering from severe exhaustion.

It is important to note that this questionnaire does not replace an expert diagnosis. However, it could be a useful start in understanding your levels of burnout. If you're concerned over your burnout level seek out an expert in healthcare.

After you've assessed how much you're burning out then you are able creating a plan of recuperation. Making a recovery strategy is a crucial step to recuperating from burnout. It will assist you determine the actions you must take to reduce your symptoms decrease stress and get back into the workforce following the burnout phase.

Determine the root causes of burnout. The first part of creating a rehabilitation plan is to pinpoint the reasons for burning out. It will allow you to understand which factors cause your stress and formulate strategies for managing those causes. Common causes for burnout are workload, lack of control, a lack of social support and an insufficient work-life balance.

Make realistic and achievable goals: Having real goals is vital to getting back from burning out. Set goals that are unrealistic can cause frustration and worsen the symptoms of burnout. Create small, achievable objectives that help feel more in satisfaction and control.

Do self-care regularly: It is essential to getting over burning out. It can involve getting adequate sleeping, eating a nutritious diet, getting involved in regular exercise and making some time to unwind and relax.

Get assistance from family, friends as well as colleagues can aid in managing the effects of burnout and gain an appreciation for social connections. You may want to consult an expert in mental health to receive additional assistance.

Stress reduction is an essential aspect of recovering from burnout, as stress is an important factor in burning out. There are a variety of strategies that can be employed to reduce stress. One strategy is to practice methods of relaxation, such as yoga, deep breathing meditation and deep breathing, all of which can will help reduce stress and help promote peace. A different strategy is to take breaks throughout the day. These breaks will help to reduce stress and improve productivity. It is essential to take short breaks to stretch, go for the stairs and breathe some fresh air or take part in a brief meditation exercise, such as deep breath or a progressive relaxation of muscles.

A break from work may help you relax as well as some time to unwind could help you feel more productive and focused before returning to working. It is possible to set alerts or reminders to the computer or smartphone so that they can take breaks throughout the working day. Also, it is recommended to incorporate longer breaks for lunch, like a break into your schedule to allow plenty of time to take a break from the work environment and recharge.

The need for support from friends and family is essential for anyone dealing with burnout. Because burnout can cause isolation and lonely, it is essential to seek help from family, friends as well as colleagues and even therapy. A person to talk to helps one be less isolated and supply individuals with aid and support needed to overcome. Self-care practices are crucial to recovering from fatigue. It involves things such as sleeping enough and eating a balanced lifestyle, engaging in regular exercising, and dedicating breaks for activities and hobbies which bring you joy. Engaging in mindfulness meditation and other methods of relaxation may aid in managing stress and reduce the symptoms of fatigue.

The setting of boundaries is an additional important method to prevent burnout becoming a problem in the near future. The process involves setting limits to your workload, saying no to jobs that aren't necessary, and taking breaks as required. It is essential to communicate clearly regarding boundaries between colleagues and the boss and adhere to the rules. In addition, it is advised to review one's goals and priorities, as burning out can be an indication that it's time to change their priorities. It is important to take time to think about what is most important to you and making the necessary adjustments such as setting goals for your career or pursuing other interests, or spending time with your loved ones could assist in stopping burning out from occurring again.

Find out any triggers that could lead to stress, for example working too much or juggling numerous tasks simultaneously Take measures to prevent the causes. It is also essential to discuss to your supervisor regarding the plan for recovery as well as any adjustments you might need. It could include changes to your work schedule or work responsibilities and also assistance from your colleagues or access to resources for mental health. Talk openly and honestly with your supervisor regarding the limitations you have and your requirements as you work to create a strategy which is beneficial for both of you. Be sure to focus on by one step at a and put your health first while you get back to your job.

The symptoms of exhaustion can become for you to handle all on your own. If you're suffering from severe signs or you feel that there is no gains in your recovery getting help from a professional is an excellent idea. A professional in mental health will aid you in determining the root of burnout, create strategies for coping, and give you help in your journey to healing.

There are many kinds of therapy that could be beneficial for people suffering from burnout. These include Cognitive-behavioral Therapy (CBT) that assists people identify and overcome destructive patterns of thought, as well as mindfulness-based therapy which is focused on enhancing present awareness and reduction of stress. Therapists can assist you in identifying any mental health problems that could contribute to your stress and formulate a strategy to address those concerns.

Self-care is a crucial aspect to regain your strength after burning out. This means looking after your body, mind as well as mentally in order to lessen anxiety and enhance overall health. These are self-care tips which can aid you in recovering from stress:

Regular exercise is proven to lower stress and increase mood. Try to do at least 30 minutes of moderate intensity exercise on a daily basis.

Make sure you eat a balanced and healthy diet. Consuming a balanced diet of fruits veggies, whole grain as well as lean proteins will help you feel healthier both mentally and physically.

Sleep enough: Insisting on enough sleep is crucial to recover from burning out. Try to get 7 to 9 hours of rest each every night.

Learn relaxation techniques such as deep breathing, gradual muscle relaxation meditation and yoga can reduce anxiety and boost mood.

Engage in activities you like Doing hobbies or other activities you love will help to relax and improve your mood mentally.

Be aware that burning out is an indicator that something is required to be changed making changes to deal with the causes could help you be happier both in your work environment and your private life.

One one year ago, I took the decision to end my drinking. When I made the decision I did not consider myself an avid drinker. However, when I look back, I see that my consumption of alcohol had grown over time, with no awareness. I was using alcohol as a way to manage in order to manage the stress that came with working in Corporate America as well as it became a habit that was challenging to quit.

In the meantime I was suffering from exhaustion from my job. Long hours, constant stress, and the constant pressure have taken their physical and mental toll on my physical wellbeing. I felt exhausted constantly, angry and constantly on edge. I knew that something had changed but didn't know what to do.

After some thought it became clear that drinking alcohol caused me to feel exhausted. This was an opportunity to ease my overwhelmed and anxiety, but it also made me feel more miserable longer-term. I decided to cut down on drinking not in order to boost my physical well-being, but also to improve my emotional and mental health.

The initial weeks were challenging. I needed to come up with different ways of dealing with anxiety and stress and I lacked drinking socially with colleagues and friends. As time went by I began to see the positive effects. I felt more energetic and was less stressed, and I was able to better handle my stress. Also, the sleeping quality increased significantly. I could focus on my job and was more productive than I had ever felt.

The decision to stop drinking gave me the ability to see why I was feeling burnt out and to take action to fix the issue. I set boundaries for myself for myself at work, stating no to jobs that were not necessary, and took break throughout my day in order to refresh. I also began to practice mindfulness meditation as well as other techniques for relaxation to reduce my anxiety. When I look back, quitting drinking was among the most beneficial choices I've made. It allowed me to recover from exhaustion and boost my overall wellbeing. Now I have more focus and focus on my work and private life. I am grateful for the positive effect it's had on my physical and mental wellbeing.

The movement of the sober curious has assisted numerous people such as me to explore the advantages of sobriety as well as take care of their health and wellbeing as a priority. The decision to stop drinking has no longer been an option that is only for people who drink; it's an individual choice that everyone can take in order to better their living.

Chapter 12: Creating a Sustainable Work-Life Balance

In the current world of speed finding a balance between work and life balance may seem like an overwhelming job. In the midst of family commitments, as well as your own goals, it can be a challenge to make sufficient time for all of it. Yet, having a healthy time-to-work balance is vital to your professional and personal success. In this article we'll discuss the significance of establishing an appropriate work-life balance. We will also look at strategies for effectively managing time and staying organized, as well as ways of making targets and managing expectations.

The ability to maintain a balanced work-life balance is vital for our well-being, both mental and physical. If we are too busy and don't take time for our own life, we are at risk of burnout as well as stress and issues with our health. However doing nothing for work could cause financial instability and stagnation in our careers. Therefore, having a balanced time-to-work balance is crucial to the health of our bodies and for our overall achievement.

Apart from the health benefits, having a good work-life balance is also able to boost our productivity as well as creative thinking. If we can unwind and recharge, we come back to work with renewed enthusiasm and a fresh perspective. This may lead to better thinking, decision-making, and problem-solving the ability to innovate.

The ability to maintain a balanced work-life balance is vital to overall health. For this to be achieved the importance of prioritizing your tasks is paramount. Begin by listing those tasks you consider the most crucial and have to be done every day. This way it will help you stay on track and stop wasting your time on things that don't matter.

Alongside prioritizing your tasks and setting goals that are realistic is essential as well. Set realistic goals for every week, day or month is a great way to remain focused and not feel overwhelmed. By breaking tasks down into smaller, manageable parts can keep you focus and prevent feeling overwhelmed.

As well as the other techniques for achieving the perfect work-life balance it's important to utilize an extensive calendar or planner. In keeping track of your all activities, both personal and professional regardless of how little they may be, on the same calendar could assist you in maintaining a clear view of all your obligations and help you avoid double-booking crucial events.

Make sure to include exact dates and hours of the events you plan to attend in your schedule to assist you in organize your schedule more effectively. Being aware of what time and place you'll need to be by a certain moment can allow you to stay clear of stress and panic at the last minute. In addition, having important details like what you need to bring or wear for an occasion will help you not have to find things you require in the nick of time.

In the process of the delegation of tasks, it's essential not just to allow time for other essential tasks but also assist in the development of other employees and create an even stronger group. If you assign tasks to someone else it is possible to not just concentrate on work that requires your unique capabilities and skills, as well as help other people develop their skills and help in the overall success of your team.

Eliminating distractions is essential in maintaining a healthy life-work equilibrium. Beware of distractions like emails, social media or meetings that are not needed. It will help you remain focus and not waste your time with non-essential tasks. Breaks throughout your day will help you keep your energy levels up and prevent burnout. You can take short breaks during the day to stretch out, take walks, or to sit down to meditate.

In the process of creating objectives and establishing expectations, the importance of being realistic. Create goals that you can achieve with the resources and time that are available. Inadequate goals could lead to anger and exhaustion. Making clear your expectations to your colleagues as well as managers and your family members can prevent misunderstandings and help manage expectations.

Understanding your limits is essential. Refraining from tasks or obligations that go beyond your capabilities can allow you to keep from feeling overwhelmed and ensure an appropriate balance between work and life. Continuously reviewing your progress towards your objectives and making adjustments to your schedule as needed can aid you in staying on the right the right track, and prevent you from wasting your hours on tasks that are not achieving your objectives.

The final step to create an effective work-life balance is about the prioritization of tasks, creating realistic goals making use of a calendar or planner and delegating work, eliminating distractions, taking time out and being sensible, dividing work into smaller chunks communication of expectations by saying no when it is necessary and regularly evaluating your progress. If you follow these tips will help you maintain a good balance between work and life and boost your overall wellbeing.

Being afraid of losing your job could be a huge stressor and cause anxiety and anxiety, particularly when you're in an outstanding debt load and have no emergency fund to draw on. A constant fear of getting dismissed can cause stress, which may adversely affect your overall health and work productivity.

If you're feeling financial strain It's crucial to take care of the financial aspects of your life along with the balance between work and life. Implementing steps to better manage your money and create the financial protection you need will help lower anxiety and stress levels as well as improve your general feeling of safety.

A way to tackle your financial burden is to set up your own budget and follow the plan. Through tracking your earnings and expenditures, you will be more aware of how much money you are spending and pinpoint areas in which you may be able to cut back. This will help you plan your spending, and also reduce amount of debt as time passes.

A fund for emergencies is a crucial way to ensure financial security. When you set aside funds in a savings account you will be able to create a security cover for sudden expenses or disruptions in income like being fired from your job.

In addition, you must take care of any concerns regarding your performance at work or in productivity which could be contributing to the fear that you could lose your job. Asking for feedback from your boss or coworkers, and taking steps to increase your capabilities and understanding can allow you to feel more secure and confident within your job.

When you take care of your personal finances and attempting to lower anxiety and stress levels, you will enhance your general feeling of safety and work productivity.

Chapter 13: Cultivating Resilience

For jobs that are high-stress Resilience is essential in maintaining healthy life-work equilibrium and to avoid burning out. Resilience means the ability to adjust and recover from setbacks difficulties, and even adversity. Here are a few strategies for creating resilience

Create a mindset of growth: Growth mindset refers to the conviction that knowledge and capabilities can be developed by hard work, commitment and persistence. Growing a mindset is able to make you see setbacks as a chance to learn and improvement. The development of a growth mindset has changed the game for me both in my personal as well as professional. Being someone who was able to be a person with a fixed outlook and a fixed mindset, I often became depressed and despair whenever faced with difficulties or obstacles. As I learned more about growing mindsets as I grew older, I started to alter my outlook and perspective on challenges.

An example of how to build an attitude of growth is to change the way you frame self-talk that is negative. Instead of thinking "I'm just not good at this" or "I'll never be able to do it," I currently say "I haven't figured it out yet, but I will keep trying." Through changing my inner dialogue I've been able to tackle challenges with more enthusiasm and willingness to continue learning.

Another method to develop an attitude of growth is to accept the possibility of failure as an opportunity to learn. The past was when I would be wary of taking chances for fear of failing. Now, I consider failing as a normal element of learning. If I experience an incident of failure, I consider, "What can I learn from this experience?" In this way, I've found myself able to recover from failures faster and have more resilience.

In the end, fostering a growth perspective is a great method of developing resilience and recovering from defeats. When we view challenges as an opportunity for improvement, we will be able to take on challenges with a optimistic and positive mindset and ultimately lead to better achievement in our personal as well as professional life.

The practice of self-care is a crucial element of gaining resilient. It is about looking after your mental, physical and emotional wellbeing in order to better deal against stress and challenges. A good way to take care of yourself is to schedule regular physical activity. Be it going for running, going to an exercise class or doing weight training, exercises will increase your energy levels, decrease the stress level, and enhance the overall quality of your wellbeing. This helps me feel more in control. an increased sense of control, and help me feel more confident to face whatever obstacles come my path.

The development of a solid support system is vital to building resilientness in the workplace of America since it allows individuals to feel less isolated and at one with others. This can be particularly important when working in stressful environments where workers may feel that they're constantly fighting against deadlines, challenging coworkers and other obstacles.

The support networks that includes family members, friends, and coworkers can serve as an opportunity to share ideas as well as help to solve problems and provide emotional support during tough moments. If, for instance, someone is facing an issue with a coworker or project is struggling, they may turn to a friend or colleague who can offer assistance or to listen. This could help ease tension and anxiety.

Establishing relationships with colleagues aids in building trust and unity in a work environment. This can help create an environment of positive workplace culture in which employees feel valued and appreciated that can boost employee satisfaction and engage.

A practical way to build an effective support system within the workplace is by arranging regularly scheduled team building events or retreats offsite. The retreats allow employees to connect with one another beyond work, and develop strong relationships that carry over into work. Another option is to identify an employee mentor to provide advice and help, specifically for those employees who might be not familiar with the organization or to the field.

Personally, I've seen the advantages of a strong community of support within the workplace. While engaged in a challenging task I was able to consult a colleague who has experience in this area for help and advice. The advice and support she provided helped me stay engaged and focused. And in the end, we managed to finish the task successfully. Furthermore, having a trusted colleague who could talk to and talk about my issues to made the task appear less overwhelming and achievable.

It can be difficult to stay optimistic particularly during tough times within Corporate America. But, keeping optimism can aid in keeping your focus and keep your focus on the goals you have set. Studies have shown that being optimistic will result in better results throughout your life such as working.

A good way to keep your optimism is to look for positive aspects in every circumstance. Through the tough times Try to think of reasons to be thankful or take away from the experiences. If, for instance, you are given negative feedback by your boss regarding a task Try to see this as an opportunity for you to increase your knowledge and skills. know-how.

Another method to keep your optimism is by surrounding your self with positive people. Surrounding yourself with positive and caring people will help keep a an optimistic outlook on your work and life. Find colleagues or acquaintances who inspire and are happy as well as try spending more time with them.

Also, it is important to develop positive self-talk. That means you should use positive words in your conversations with yourself in moments of anxiety or stress. Instead of saying "I can't do this" or "this is too difficult," think of saying something like "I can handle this" or "I'm capable of overcoming this challenge."

Furthermore, setting reasonable and achievable goals will make you more optimistic. If you accomplish any goal, no matter what size, it will bring you feelings of satisfaction and inspire your to keep working toward the bigger goals.

Staying positive is crucial to build resilience in corporate America. Focusing on the positives, surrounded with people who are positive, using positive self-talk and setting achievable goals and goals, you can keep an optimistic outlook on working and your life in the midst of difficult moments. Apart from building resilient, it's essential to remain focused and motivated in difficult situations.

Recognizing your achievements regardless of how modest they are, is an effective way to boost the motivation of your attention. Recognition of your accomplishments and accomplishments towards your goals can aid you in staying on the right course and gain momentum toward greater successes. This is especially helpful after a bout of burnout since it's difficult to not get caught up by feelings of anxiety or disappointment.

An effective method to celebrate accomplishments is to look back at your accomplishments. It could be as simple as writing down your accomplishments and sharing your accomplishments to a friend or loved ones, or acknowledging your achievements and offer you a hug on your back. It is important to keep in mind that every move you take regardless of how tiny it may seem, is an important step toward the proper direction.

A second way to acknowledge the achievements you have made is to give yourself a reward to acknowledge your efforts. This can be as simple as letting yourself indulge in an indulgence in a favourite snack or engaging with a soothing activity for example, a massage or even a night out with a film. Set up a reward program is a great and efficient way of keeping your mind and body engaged during the process of recovery.

The final step is to celebrate your accomplishments. This may also include the sharing of your experiences with others. It doesn't matter if you're part of an organization that supports you, a recovery program or even the sober-minded group, telling your achievements by sharing them with other people can make you feel more connected, encouraged and energized. You can also help others who are facing similar struggles.

Keep in mind that celebrating your accomplishments does not mean that you have to be the best or doing everything simultaneously. It's about celebrating your accomplishments as well as staying committed and gaining momentum toward the goals you have set. Therefore, take time to be proud of your accomplishments however small you may consider them, and make use of them to fuel you in going forward toward recuperation.

Being flexible is an important part of regaining your energy after burnout. Remember that unexpected obstacles and setbacks could occur so being able to adjust and adapt your plan accordingly could help on your journey to recovery. Flexibility means being open to new concepts and methods, even though they differ from the plan you originally had. Also, it means having the ability to adjust your strategy in the event that something isn't working.

The best way to be flexible is to maintain your mind open and willing to hear feedback from other people. Inquiring about comments from friends, colleagues as well as a therapist may offer valuable information on how you can make your life more efficient and reduce stress. Remember that feedback isn't a form of criticism but rather it's an opportunity to improve.

Furthermore, being flexible could require rethinking your priorities and goals throughout the process of recovery. When you acquire new knowledge and new perspectives, you could realize that the things you once considered essential to you could have no meaning or important. The ability to adjust the goals and priorities you set helps you to stay in line with the things that matter to you. It can also prevent the possibility of burnout at some point in the future.

Also, being flexible implies being gentle with your self and accepting a degree of failure. There is a normal tendency to face some setbacks, or even days when you're not feeling more productive or focused than you'd would like. Instead of blaming yourself instead, you should take these situations with love and enthusiasm. Consider what you could take away from this experience and then utilize it as an opportunity to grow and growth. Be aware that recovering from burnout can be a long-distance journey which is why being flexible and agile can aid you through your way through the ups and downs on your journey.

The bottom line is that building resilience, and remaining focus and motivated during tough situations is vital to maintain an appropriate work-life balance as well as avoid burning out. Develop an effective support system be optimistic and establish goals and plans to reach these goals. Be flexible and be happy with the achievements, no matter what they are, in order to keep your enthusiasm and keep you focused.

Chapter 14: Finding Joy and Purpose

Your Work Many of us jobs consume an enormous amount of our energy and time. It is difficult to get stuck in working routines, tired and unfulfilled by the work we do. Finding joy and motivation in what you do is vital to general well-being and productivity. It is also helpful to think about the reasons you decided on this profession to begin with. Spend some time reflecting on the things that made you feel satisfied and happy throughout your career and what you could do to get the same feeling. In this article we'll explore methods to find meaning and fulfillment throughout your professional life.

Finding your values' core and goals is an essential approach to finding happiness and meaning in the work you do no matter if you're within Corporate America or any other sector. When you consider what is the your most significant thing as a person and what drives you, you will discover what your job can do to match your ideals and goals.

If, for instance, you're interested in social justice issues and social justice, you could find joy by a job where you can work toward bringing about positive social change. In contrast when personal development is important to your life, you might be able to find fulfillment in a job which offers the opportunity to learn and advancement.

After you've identified your primary values and the reason for being It is important to discover ways to align your activities to reflect these ideals. It could mean looking for assignments or projects that are aligned with your beliefs and figuring out ways to integrate the values you hold dear into your schedule.

In the world of corporate America the quest for fulfillment and joy at work is hard, especially within a highly high-stakes and fast-paced work working environment. By focusing on your beliefs and goals and focusing on your core values, you will be able to generate a sense of purpose and happiness in your work that can result in more satisfaction in your job and a better overall wellbeing.

In addition, you should look for opportunities to grow and advancement in your professional career regardless of whether it's by way of mentorship, training programs and pursuing fresh problems. Through continuous learning and development within your profession it is possible to remain active and enthusiastic, as well as find more enjoyment and fulfillment in your job.

Then, think about the purpose of your the world. What goals do you hope to accomplish with your work and how do you align it with your own beliefs? Once you've got a solid knowledge of your primary goals and values that you are able to better focus your efforts on the things that matter to you most.

Recall why you picked your profession initially. Was there something that made you feel enthusiastic about the work you did when you first started? At times, we get distracted from the passion we have for and enthusiasm that drives us to the work we do as we become caught up in routines and anxiety.

Remember when you started your career within your area. Which were the things you enjoyed most? What aspects of your job provide you with the highest satisfaction? Find ways to connect to those areas. If you are interested by helping other people, think about taking on a mentorship role or volunteering in a cause that is related to the field you work in. If you like solving complicated issues, you should look for interesting challenges, or consider taking on projects that are not your normal duties. If you're a believer in the ability to think outside of the box, search for ways to introduce innovative ideas to your group.

It's equally important to ensure that your job is aligned to your values, core beliefs and mission. If your job does not match what you are, it may be difficult to achieve fulfillment. Think about whether the current organization and job description aligns to your own values and the changes you could do to ensure that your career is in line in line with your mission.

Work isn't necessarily an obsession to have meaning and a reason behind it. A lot of people are satisfied just doing their job well in their workplace and helping to ensure its achievement. In the seemingly insignificant business of Corporate America There are many opportunities for making an contribution to the success of your company.

A way to be more purposeful within your job is to concentrate on the impact that your business makes to the world. A lot of successful companies have committed to a socially responsible corporate governance approach and take steps to decrease their carbon footprint and give back to their local communities. If you can align your values to the mission of your business it is possible to feel satisfaction by knowing you're striving for a better world.

Another method to make sense when working in a Corporate America work is to utilize your time off to engage with community or charitable work. A lot of companies offer volunteering opportunities, or help with employee-led initiatives. Utilizing your talents and abilities to aid others, you will achieve your goals and feel fulfilled beyond the office.

The key to find joy and meaning within your job is to make it aligned with your ideals and values. If you are able to find joy in the process itself or its impact in the world, it's crucial to remain true to your values and what drives you. When you do this you will find purpose and satisfaction even in those tasks that seem to be the least important.

A positive outlook helps you to find happiness and motivation in your job. Instead of dwelling on the negative elements of your job you should try to change your perspective to look at things that are positive. Discover ways to be grateful for your challenges and the possibilities which come from your work. Be focused on the skills you could discover and the ways you can develop.

Be grateful by reminiscing about the things you're grateful for at work. Recognize your accomplishments and those of your coworkers. Through cultivating a positive outlook it will improve the quality of your life and perform better in your work.

Growing your skill set can be an effective way to gain satisfaction and meaning within your job. If, for instance, you're in the field of finance and you are interested in enrolling into a program to understand more about investing sustainably, which could align with your beliefs and allow you to get more satisfaction from your job. For those who work in the field of marketing, you might undertake a project which requires you to learn the field of social media marketing as well as graphic design.

Learn new techniques can improve your self-confidence in the job you do. In the case of trying to learn the latest software attending a training course or attending a class could help you develop the knowledge you require to become more effective and efficient in the work you do. Also, learning new techniques could help you be noticed at work and prepare your self for advancement or jobs.

The ability to expand your knowledge can enable you to investigate new careers or fields. In the case of example, if you are in the medical industry it is possible to study a degree in healthcare administration in order to discover potential opportunities in management. If you're in the tech industry and are interested into a program in artificial intelligence or machine learning in order to discover possible new avenues in this field.

In the end, improving your skills will help you feel more fulfilled and fulfillment in your job as it allows you to expand as a person, develop, and progress within your profession. Also, take advantage of opportunities to increase your understanding and skills, and remain willing to take on the possibilities of new challenges.

Another way to experience fulfillment and joy within your job is to develop positive relationships with your colleagues, clients or clients. This could mean looking for ways to work with other people for projects or ideas and also establishing the foundation of a community that is supportive within your work environment.

Working closely with colleagues and working with them, you will gain fresh perspective on your work, as well as learn from their own experiences. It can allow you to grow professionally and personally and make your work more enjoyable as well as rewarding.

As well as working closely with coworkers, it's essential to build strong connections with customers or clients. Through providing excellent customer service and establishing strong bonds to those who you interact with it will help you create a sense of purpose and significance in your job.

The development of positive relationships at the workplace also helps in reducing stress levels and improving your overall health. If you are feeling supported and bonded to the people in the workplace, you're more likely to feel happy and content in your work.

In order to build relationships that are positive It is essential to be friendly and open as well as actively listening to those around you. Look for opportunities to network to others by taking part in networking events and gatherings with friends, and spend the time to familiar with your colleagues on a an individual scale.

It is also crucial to cultivate compassion and empathy as you interact with other people. If you can put yourself in who is not you and examining the perspective of others, you will be able to improve your relationships with others and build the perfect work environment.

In the end, building interactions in the workplace can be a major influence on your overall health and importance in the work you do. If you are looking for ways to work together and communicate with other people, you will make a positive community and experience greater satisfaction within your work.

Alongside finding happiness and fulfillment in the work you do but it's also essential to be able to find fulfillment outside of the work you do. Engaging in hobbies and pursuits in other areas of life can allow you to live a more balanced life and feel more fulfilled all-around. If it's playing a game or painting, gardening or cooking, choose what you enjoy to do and then put time and effort in the activity.

The ability to connect with friends and family is also vital to find something meaningful in life outside of working. Spend time with your beloved people, whether that's eating meals together, planning an excursion on a weekend or just chatting via the phone. The connections you make can create the feeling of belonging and connection that is extremely satisfying.

Be aware that if you lead a an enjoyable life in addition to work, it will help your professional life. Participating in the activities and relationships which bring joy and fulfillment will give you the drive and enthusiasm to tackle your job with more enthusiasm and originality. Additionally, it can help an understanding and balance required to face the stress and challenges of working.

Chapter 15: Get Clarity Success, Different

Every day, you get up. It could be early at dawn, or it could be during an event or a meeting, but you'll. When you wake up, you'll know that the success stories which surround you aren't the kind of things you would like for yourself.

It's a sensation that fades away. If you're anything like me, it's likely that you'll move the line of goal once you're close. How can we move towards achieving a goal that's true to us as people?

Reminisce about times when you had success when you were a kid. Which memories come to mind? It's when I hear the praise of an artwork I was particularly happy with or even for something that was a bit silly like guessing how many gumballs contained in the container. Also, I remember being cheered by people who were successful in getting high marks or for tidying up my space--things which didn't matter any to me, yet seemed significant to other people. The habit of doing more pleasing others becomes an ingrained habit in us when we get older. Our inner voice, which yells that we should do the things we love is drowned out by the joyful voices of those we've admired which is why we go all-in on the things that earned us the praise of others.

There is a very small chance that someone in your workplace, whether a coworker or parent can see that you are doing something right, or putting in the effort and then ask "Is that really what you wanted?" The majority of the time, they react with excitement, appreciation or thanks. Montessori school models stress choice--"Choose the work you do" is the motto for the school's curriculum. However, this is a rare exception and isn't a norm after you've graduated from the school system and entering a job position. Yes, you may offer to take on more duties, but employers aren't usually equipped to accept these requests from determined employees. They're there to assist to complete your job effectively.

Your only source of guidance for your success. It is up to you to decide your own goals and what you want to accomplish. It can be very challenging to distinguish from your life in general So I'd suggest looking at some categories as you try to revise your own personal definition.

TRY

Success--today's definition

The time has come to refresh your words to describe the goals you've set and the reason you work hard for each day.

Think about these common elements of the definition of success. Which of these, if you can, are you defining as "success" today? Be honest with yourself and observe what's real.

Take up to 10 minutes to describe these types of categories.

The place you reside

Size, location and type of the house

Facilities on-site or close by

You can buy what you need regularly effortlessly

Entertainment, food, clothes, and entertainment

What is the frequency of replacing objects; how expensive are they?

The autonomy of your time

What is the average number of hours you have to work every day or every week?

Who determines if the job is done well, properly, enough?

The relationships you cherish

Do you have a person that you enjoy spending time with? Few/many?

Which are the deepest and the breadths of these bonds?

You have the authority to exercise it

A leader, expert and person of authority, and a and a trusted

In the next step, highlight or circle the words that make you think - what is a fact that's incredibly true. Incorporate new words as they pop into your head. Copy the most powerful, authentic words onto the sections below.

Then, set a clock for 10 minutes, and think about each sentence or word that you have read. Remember the origin of the truth. Where you gained the ambition to achieve the success.

Who has praised you? Who do you mimic?

What action or project has earned the praise?

Do you remember some of your personal feelings concerning it before the effort or result was noticed by another person?

Do you think you would be happy If your accomplishment was kept secret for the rest of your existence?

After this, if you'd like to change or improve a couple of your phrases, you can take action.

Then, narrow the list down to just five words - your updated definition of success.

1

2

3

4

5

Put them up where you'll notice them in the day. Bonus points if they're located in an accessible location which you can see them throughout the entire day. I've captured a photograph of mine and put it on the lock screen of my mobile devices to ensure that I can see the screen often.

They are your own and important, up-to-date definition of what it means to be successful. It is the reason you strive above and beyond to satisfy your requirements. You can use them to improve the tasks you concentrate on professionally, what tasks you undertake, and who you want to collaborate with closely. Take note of the many methods throughout the day that you're encouraged to pursue the different kinds of successes.

Achieving success for you could translate to money in the six figures or a new home or more prestigious titles. The success of someone else could be controlling their work schedule and having the time to take care for their loved ones and having enough cash for the local community's needs. What's important is that what you're looking for should be something that can please you, not your teachers, parents or coworkers. You'll do it even there was no way anyone else could tell that you're doing it.

What is the reason your definition should be that personal?

Motivation that is intrinsically driven is what you're looking for that is the motivation to accomplish things in a way that delights you.

satisfaction comes your way regardless of the way it is thought of by others. It is different from external rewards like the praise of your boss. Individuals who are motivated by their own intrinsically aren't dependent on a great company and managers, or even supportive friends to achieve their goals. Although their voice may be more loud than it is at the moment, everyone could turn up their own level.

To increase the intrinsic motivation of your heart, it's best to begin small even though it might feel a bit silly. Don't be afraid to try it.

Make sure you turn it up to the max.

If you want your intuition to speak to you, you must pay attention. For those who are a regular crowd-pleaser, it will take time to develop into a more powerful sense of.

TRY

You can tune into your internal navigational system

Begin by going for a just a few minutes of walking. Put away the electronics and get out of the house. If you come to the point of turning, choose the direction that feels comfortable. When you reach an intersection, and after couple of breaths, you aren't able to decide the direction you'd like to go then just change direction and attempt another time at the next intersection. This exercise will show your body that it's making an effort to be attentive to it. It will also show that the body is in charge at times and not continually demanding your performance. Listening to the things you'd like to achieve when you're in a low-risk situation, like walking through your neighborhood or home will help you become familiar with how the physical sensations of your body may signal instincts towards your brain. If you practice it at this, you'll know how to stop before you send an email or agreeing to an undertaking for a moment, and observe your own desires instead of rushing in to be influenced by the other person's idea of successful.

We Are More Than Work

More than just your job.

The danger of letting the work you do become your primary image is laid out very early in our lives. "What do you want to be when you grow up?" is a common one, which has the response that you'll become what you want to be.

The advice is frequently to turn our passion into a profession, and to pursue the sake of a cause. But, I've observed that people who work on behalf of a cause or within their areas of expertise tend to be the most vulnerable to burnout and career relapse which is followed by severe depression. It is interesting to pursue your passions because you have a limited capacity to develop in them. they require long-term commitment and dedication. There's no quick way for pursuing your interest. The passion often manifests while you strive for the goal, pulling closer and further into an area or system. This isn't a collection of skills to acquire and learn, but rather a lifetime quest that guides you through the rest of your time of your day.

Chapter 16: Who Are Curious Are Fascinating?

In terms of earning from a financial perspective, being extremely curious about essential skills relevant to your professional career is crucial. While applying the same amount of attention to various different subjects makes you more multi-faceted. Prior to the time when work was all-consuming over the past 20 years that was driven mainly by a culture that was always on the tech industry It was normal and even expected that you had other pursuits to explore in your spare time. For people who haven't worked like this, your it's what happens prior to breakfast, and then after the late afternoon. The hobbies or activities could be spent in solitude or with friends. There were chess clubs or leagues for slow-pitch, prepared extravagant meals, or training in the martial arts or cycling. Musicians played solo or as part of jam bands and maybe wrote songs. Our lives were filled with interests that often gave us more energy and greater circle of connections.

Modern jobs demand more of our time that a traditional 9-to-5 job would. It is acknowledged as heroic, and even lauded.

How can you devote less effort to your job when you are not working? Find something to do that will are interesting to you!

Paint Softball Pickle ball

Martial art Biking Small engines

Drones Baking Ceramics

Volunteering Yoga Gardening

Animal training Astrology Spiritual practices

Conservation Chess Social games

Stories in a foreign language.

Computer skills Poetry

A Bit on Burnout

The wise's words

A conversation with Paloma Medina

Paloma Medina is a presenter, trainer an entrepreneur, coach and coach. Her research focuses on the neuroscience and science of life and work particularly how we can create healthy, positive workplaces and teams. Paloma has an Masters of the field of Public Administration at New York University with a concentration in applied psychology as well as improving organizational performance.

What brought you to be fascinated by the brains of your colleagues?

I returned to graduate college after I began my professional career. To admit it, I did not make the grade. Students were working the equivalent of seven or more hours per day and I couldn't concentrate on that level. I thought to myself that I might not need to be, I could do it in a different manner...

The brain has two major system: the limbic is responsible for all the essentials-- breath, heartbeat and reflexes, and so on; the other is the prefrontal cortex (PFC) which is the rational brain, which performs math or follows the Google Map route. The PFC is often tired, whereas the limbic brain is more energy and can process very fast taking quick and decisive choices. This is necessary for evolutionary progress. This is the brain that we have since our earliest days. After I was taught that, I thought, "Could my limbic brain know that there's a better way to achieve this task, if my rational brain just got out of the way?" So, the solution is "Maybe?"

Is there a case where that our brains rationality isn't able to comprehend?

Ha! What's the average number of hours do I have to be working. This is old information as well, dating back to the time when jobs were automated, and not about knowing. The typical American is employed for forty-seven hours per week. So reducing hours appears to be the "rational" win here, isn't it? Well, hours don't matter. Contrary to what you might think. are.

Are you saying that certain time is "worth more" than others?

Yes! The brain I have at 9am is completely different from my brain when I go to bed at 3pm. People are aware of this however, we tend to ignore the signals. Once I know how different my brain functions and how it functions, I am able to use my time in the morning for higher-level cognitively demanding work (when my brain's PFC isn't quite exhausted) while putting off simpler work for later in the day (when my brain is more likely to feel fatigued, i.e., feeling overwhelmed by my brain).

Cognitive overload is a term that's remarkably familiar Can you guide me through the process?

Cognitive overload occurs an issue when we do not let our PFC to relax and continue to push it to perform work, check an email, scroll through across social media, and to multitask and so on. But, the PFC similar to muscles, isn't able to be stretched beyond a specific threshold. It requires rest between to replenish. One thing I've discovered is that all of us must learn to properly take PFC breaks in order to prevent over-thinking. My first move was to note which of my activities caused me stress to my PFC (checking Instagram, for certain) and what felt like genuine restful times (lying on the floor in a closed position or listening to music). After that, I needed to consider ways to build in to protect my rest periods.

How do you know how to speak with your colleagues or even your boss regarding your requirements?

It is possible to start from at the point where you are able to go, even without having a conversation with anybody. Be careful not to be depressed regarding this. There's a tendency to think that if you cannot create big chunks of unbroken work and you're caught up. There's no such thing as all or nothing.

As I was first beginning to rethink my boundaries, I could not discover any period from 9 a.m. between 6 p.m. I felt confident asking for. I was assuming that I would not achieve it since I didn't feel comfortable asking for it, I just was not yet ready. Then I wondered "When can I squeeze in time for myself?" I thought that a time of 8:30 to 9 a.m. in the coffee shop would be a good time for me to claim it as my own time. I almost shattered myself thinking that 30 minutes was not enough. Yet I began anyway.

The first thing I noticed was that I didn't think in the similar way when I was on a packed subway like I did in a quiet spot with a cup of coffee. It was a very nourishing experience. Then, 30 became 45 minutes. I needed to wake up earlier, which at first was difficult but, it turns out to be achievable. I was able to cut off about two to three hours per week like this, which is close to my work schedules that were a bit crammed.

Be consistent versus an extended period of time. You would like to develop a routine. It's much more beneficial to take thirty minutes every day of the week rather than four hours each two weeks. Making time to get up earlier was a challenge as I had to conquer all sorts of perceived obstacles. Getting up early only on certain days really was difficult. It was a challenge to convince my husband to go out with the dog (which was his agreement, but I had assumed that it would cause a problem). Even small changes may be difficult to implement into place, but they are important to do.

People whose time limits you admire about their methods of doing it. At first, when I observed those I admired I assumed they got to do as they did because of their circumstances--seniority or autonomy. When I began to shadow their actions, it was clear for me that the majority instances of their lives were due to the fact that they had requested what they wanted.

In the end, if I've stated an opinion and requested the flexibility to come up with an agreement that is beneficial to the entire group, I've never been met with the "no." The fear of having to talk about it is usually more significant than any rejection that you may (and generally never) have to face.

Are you able to offer any suggestions for someone who's nearing their breakthrough?

The experience itself is unforgettable. Keep the fact that many people are trained for marathons. The fact is that running 26.2-miles without having trained is a disaster. 26.2-mile race without training in any way will result in injury, not only with sore muscles. It's similar to taking your toothbrush to the dentist--you could brush every day twice to a total time of four minutes or at least 28 minutes a week. But you'll have different results from both of these approaches. Remember that you need to master some regular or daily routines that allow you to take a break, instead of just running the run in Day One. Embrace smaller experiments. Take a bit of relaxation time within your daily plan. Begin by taking the day free with a purpose.